Advance Praise for

THE ECO-FOODS GUIDE

Cynthia Barstow takes us on her journey to discover that the more we know about the implications of our food choices, the healthier and freer we feel and become. We owe her a hearty "thank you" for helping to keep us awake — for offering invaluable guidance in choosing food that is satisfying to our senses and best for the Earth at the same time. She helps us choose not only the health and enjoyment we each want from eating well, but the world we want, too.

— Frances Moore Lappé, author of *Hope's Edge: The Next Diet for a Small Planet*

At last, all of the vital information I need as a food shopper is gathered together into one easy-to-use book! *The Eco-Foods Guide* is destined to become the essential companion for everyone trying to make shopping decisions that will protect both people and the planet.

— Mark Ritchie, President, Institute for Agriculture and Trade Policy

This is a truly informative book, written in a warm, personal voice, with humor, passion, and vision. There is so much confusion about food choices, even among the best-intentioned of us who would like our lifestyles to reflect our values. *The Eco-Foods Guide* is an important handbook that will walk us intelligently through the maze.

— Mollie Katzen, author of *Moosewood Cookbook* and *Sunlight Café*

Consumers need to realize that every time they shop, or sit down to eat, they're casting their vote for the kind of food system we have. Read this book. It'll help you cast your food vote for a sustainable and healthy future.

— Ronnie Cummins, National Director, Organic Consumers Association
www.organicconsumers.org

THE
ECO-FOODS
GUIDE

What's Good for
the Earth is
Good for You!

Cynthia Barstow
Foreword by Frances Moore Lappé

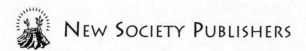
NEW SOCIETY PUBLISHERS

Cataloguing in Publication Data:

A catalog record for this publication is available from the National Library of Canada.

Cover design by Diane McIntosh. Cover image <plus ART/PHOTO NAME>

Printed in Canada by Transcontinental Printing.

New Society Publishers acknowledges the support of the Government of Canada through the Book Publishing Industry Development Program (BPIDP) for our publishing activities.

Paperback ISBN: 0-86571-460-6

Inquiries regarding requests to reprint all or part of *The Eco-Foods Guide* should be addressed to New Society Publishers at the address below. To order directly from the publishers, please add $4.50 shipping to the price of the first copy, and $1.00 for each additional copy (plus GST in Canada). Send check or money order to:

New Society Publishers
P.O. Box 189, Gabriola Island, BC V0R 1X0, Canada
1 (800) 567·6772

New Society Publishers' mission is to publish books that contribute in fundamental ways to building an ecologically sustainable and just society, and to do so with the least possible impact on the environment, in a manner that models this vision. We are committed to doing this not just through education, but through action. We are acting on our commitment to the world's remaining ancient forests by phasing out our paper supply from ancient forests worldwide. This book is one step towards ending global deforestation and climate change. It is printed on acid-free paper that is 100% old growth forest-free (100% post-consumer recycled), processed chlorine free, and printed with vegetable based, low VOC inks. For further information, or to browse our full list of books and purchase securely, visit our website at: www.newsociety.com

NEW SOCIETY PUBLISHERS

www.newsociety.com

This book is dedicated to
Emily and Willy,
who remind me
(a cappella, in unison),
*"We are the world … we are the ones who
make a brighter day, so let's start giving!"*

Table of Contents

Acknowledgments

I F NOT FOR MY IMMEDIATE SUPPORT GROUP, a handful of people who researched, read, edited, and groused with me over every detail, there would be no book. Thank you to Sarah Kelley, my assistant and researcher extraordinaire; Kathy Ruhf, my sustainable-agriculture-community editor and friend; Bonnie Emmons, my target-market editor and generous cousin; Ann Paulsen, my official and patient editor; and Lee Barstow, my most loving editor and computer relief.

Thank you to my colleagues at UMass, especially Lyle Craker and Zoë Gardner, Ed McGlew, Beth Blanchett, Nancy Garrabrants, and all my students who have been there to urge me forward. Thanks also to the many friends in the sustainable agriculture community who have either shared with me, reviewed chapters/sections, or who have been there for me throughout the process, including Michael Appleby, Annie Cheatham, Kate Clancy, Bill Coli, Jeff Dlott, Katherine DiMatteo, Randy Duckworth, Tom Green, Joan Gussow, Hal Hamilton, Deborah Kane, Dan Kaplan, David Kline, Ruth Katz, Bruce Mertz, Fran McManus, Tod Murphy, Ron Prokopy, Carolyn Raffensperger, Mark Ritchie, Francine Stephens, Liz Wheeler, Glenda Yoder, and Don Zasada, all the Brookfield Board members, the NESAWG steering committee members, and all the people I have missed who should be acknowledged here.

I also want to thank my children, Emily, Willy, and Taylor, for hanging in there; my parents, Bill and Nancy Miller, for their love and encouragement; and the Stonecliffe contingent, for their support. Thank you to my publisher, Chris Plant, for his enthusiasm and support throughout the process. To Linda Roghaar, who is not only my agent, but so much more, thank you for everything you do for me , and for that one magical moment when you said, "Hey, you have a book here!"

Finally, and most importantly, thank you to my husband, Lee, my spiritual partner who keeps me grounded and never fails to show up for me, every single day.

Foreword
by Frances Moore Lappé

MIGHT CYNTHIA BARSTOW'S VERY TERM "ECO-FOODS" CAUSE SOME TO RESPOND, "What? You mean I should make eating some kind of statement? Please, just let me enjoy food, don't ask me to think about it!" Over the years, I've met any number of people who bristle at the notion of basing our food choices on anything other than taste. It will diminish enjoyment, they believe.

For me, though, it's been a lifetime of discovering that the more I choose food based on the effects of my choices, the more pleasure I get from eating. The more I act on what I know, the less I feel like a victim, and the more power I feel I have. Knowledge has changed me, but has not destroyed enjoyment. In fact, I've learned that knowledge greatly improves taste. Thus, *The Eco-Foods Guide* can be viewed as a flavor enhancer.

We might think that consciously choosing what we eat is somehow "political" — and of course it is. However, the most important food choice a person can make in today's world is not whether to buy organic or locally grown food, or whether to avoid meat or genetically modified food; it's choosing to walk into a fast-food chain or grabbing processed food off the supermarket shelf. These actions say a great deal more than one would think; they reinforce a particular structure of decision-making power in our society, one that undermines our own well-being. A typical American supermarket sells 30,000 different items, half of which are produced by a mere ten corporations. And on the boards of these ten corporations sit 138 people, a tiny group deciding what goes into our bodies. Now that's power!

An epidemic is sweeping this country. The epidemic is obesity: now six in ten adults are overweight or obese. In defining the epidemic as obesity, however, we can mislead ourselves: Obesity is a result, not a cause. The main problem is the food we're eating — the high-fat, salty, sugar-laden, processed, meat-centered diet, unknown to our species until this generation. This food is fueling not only heart disease and cancer, but diabetes, hypertension, and other life-threatening illness.

Some argue that people have the right to choose food that's bad for them. But choice requires no coercion, and real options, as well as awareness of the consequences — all sadly lacking. A species choosing to eat what's literally killing it would certainly be an evolutionary first!

In our schools, too, choice is narrowing. More than half of the California schools surveyed recently serve branded foods. Hundreds of school districts have signed "pouring rights" contracts to sell only one soft-drink company's brand. (Even one additional soft drink a day may increase a child's obesity risk by as much as 60 percent.) Schools now sell $750 million in junk food from vending machines each year. This, even though childhood obesity has doubled in the last 20 years.

It's no mystery why food companies are able to push their products so easily. Human beings evolved with what nutritionists call a "weak satiation" mechanism for sugar and fat — meaning we can eat a lot at one time — because this trait served us well as hunter-gatherers. Now it's our Achilles' heel, and food companies have us by that heel. Half the calories Americans consume now come from fat and sugar.

Our choices are even more constricted because institutions, entrusted with helping us sort out what's healthy and what's not (including the US Department of Agriculture), are themselves influenced by lobbyists within the food industry. But consumers are beginning to rebel. The USDA was recently found, in a suit launched by the Washington-based Physicians Committee for Responsible Medicine, to have stacked a panel that evaluates the nation's food guidelines with representatives from the meat and dairy industry. And now some educators and parents have realized that fast food in schools is almost as dangerous as cigarettes; at least 20 states have introduced bills to limit low-nutrition foods in schools.

Beyond schools, each of us can participate. We can choose to simply not respond to food industry propaganda (i.e., advertising). Our single most important choice might well be where we shop for food. If we forego supermarkets as much as possible and connect with community-supported agriculture, linking us directly with local organic farms in the summer, and if we shop in food co-ops and farmers' markets, our palates are consistently tempted by precisely the whole plant foods best for our bodies. If we demand public policies that shift tax subsidies away from large chemical operations and toward independent family and non-chemical farms, we make choosing healthy food easier for all of us.

Cynthia Barstow takes us on her journey to discover that the more we know about the implications of our food choices, the healthier and freer we feel and become. We owe her a hearty "thank you" for helping to keep us awake — for offering invaluable guidance in choosing food that is satisfying to our senses and best for the Earth at the same time. She helps us choose not only the health and enjoyment we each want from eating well, but the world we want, too.

Introduction

I FELT LIKE A SCHOOLGIRL AGAIN, STRETCHING MY ARM TOWARD THE CEILING, hoping to be called upon. The prominent soil scientist at the University of Massachusetts had just finished his lecture about the importance of environmental conservation of soils. All the graduate students were shooting off questions about blue-green algae and other advanced subjects; I simply wanted to know about the effects of lime on my garden. His response to my question was one of rather dismissive impatience. I continued, "But the point I'm trying to make, sir, is that as a consumer, I don't know what is good for the Earth … and if something is not good for the Earth, how can it be good for me?" He moved on to the really important topics.

That experience is one of many I had when I first fell in love with the subject of food and the Earth, which got under my skin and, like an itch, continued to draw my attention toward our disconnection between what we eat and where it grows. In the early days, the professor's response was typical. Many in the world of academic agriculture dismissed the uninformed eater as ignorant and "out of their league." Today many more experts are beginning to acknowledge the importance of our eating habits to the environmental health of our planet.

For most of my life, I ate without a single thought about where the food came from. As a child, I had learned to garden with my grandfather and to grow cherry tomatoes with my mom. Since then, I had never had soil under my nails from nurturing a plant. By the time I was 30, I was vice-president of marketing for a $3-billion restaurant company in Manhattan, selling fast food in low-income neighborhoods and cheap food in high-priced tourist areas. I knew I was allowing some serious buildup of negative karma. Thankfully, it didn't last long.

My husband and I left Manhattan to start a family in Amherst, Massachusetts. When we first arrived, we lived in a house surrounded by a beautiful apple orchard. Unfortunately, the trees were sprayed continuously with noxious agricultural chemicals. A neighboring farmer would arrive in a yellow slicker and hat and carrying a huge nozzle. I would rush around, trying to catch our dog, to get into the house as quickly as possible to reduce my chances of exposure. The dissonance was growing. Trying to create a new life while avoiding pesticide spray every few days was disturbing, to say the least.

At the same time, I began my first garden since childhood. I wanted to savor the flavors of foods grown by my own hand — to experience that unique connection with what I was eating. With several gardening books under my arm and questions aplenty, I bombarded our local nursery with questions. Unfortunately, the nursery staff had just as many to send back my way. What about inoculated seeds? Did I want bone meal or chemical fertilizer? I was lost, and the agitation continued. What would these things do to my precious vegetables? That special relationship I was hoping to cultivate seemed doomed. I didn't know enough, but I knew something was wrong.

It was then that the sustainable agriculture bug bit me. Deciding not to pontificate without substance and to learn enough to grow a plant, I enrolled in the Stockbridge School of Agriculture to study fruits and vegetables. At this point, someone gave me a copy of the 20th anniversary edition of *Diet for a Small Planet* by Frances Moore Lappé. Here was a book that gave solutions and expressed many of the frustrations I had been having about our food system ... and it spoke to the consumer! The author kept referring to the responsibility we all share to change how we eat and ultimately to protect the Earth. The constant discomfort I had been feeling was starting to lessen — there were answers, individually and collectively.

> **"I never met a person who didn't care about our environment or didn't think it important to keep the Earth healthy for future generations. Most people want to contribute to the solution."**

Since then, I have been fortunate to work with many growers, agriculture students, and consumer groups. I have spent a great deal of time trying to learn as much as possible about why people might be interested in eco-foods. I learned that people really care about buying foods that are good for the Earth and good for their health. As Lappé said, "Another part of the good news ... is that what's good for the Earth is good for us, too."[1]

In all the study and focus groups I took part in, I never met a person who didn't care about our environment or didn't think it important to keep the Earth healthy for future generations. Most people want to contribute to the solution. For some, it has become a way of life. For others, it has become like a gnat, a perpetual "gotta-do-that," that flies around the grocery store with every visit.

Anecdotal information from other mothers has been incredibly valuable. From winter book clubs to summer moms'-night-out potlucks, I have heard what seems to be a universal frustration with what to buy at the grocery store. "How bad is rBGH?" one friend will ask. "Is salmon back on the okay-to-eat list?" from another. Food shoppers seem to be in a quandary. They want healthy, wholesome, good-for-the-Earth food, but they don't want to spend their whole lives learning what is on the okay list.

I have written this guide to serve this audience. It will not be complete enough for advocates steeped in farm politics; it will not be scientific enough for the academic hoping to learn the most recent discoveries in biotechnology. This book is for those who want to learn enough to inform their shopping decisions, to start them off on a path of discovery and involvement.

This book attempts to simplify extremely complex issues without being superficial. The information I share is just the tip of the iceberg — an entry point into an agricultural system in need of recovery, and an introduction to the people and projects that make up its support group.

This book contains many personal reflections and opinions. It is important to me to maintain a conversational style. I am not an investigative reporter; I am a working mom who has landed in the midst of a wonderful movement toward a sustainable food system. I want to share it in the best way I can … by inviting you to join me in the grocery aisles and out in the fields.

In an article in the *Denver Post* a few months ago, a reporter wrote, "Traditional links between Americans and the soil, seeds, and sun that sustain us has been cut off like a sheet of Saran Wrap."[2]

> "We deserve to know more about our foods and how they were grown or raised, so that our everyday meals move from catch-what-you-can to a communion with nature."

We deserve to know more about our foods and how they were grown or raised, so that our everyday meals move from catch-what-you-can to a communion with nature. Ultimately, we need this journey because "what is good for the Earth, is good for you." I hope *The Eco-Foods Guide* will be a start.

Shopping for Eco-foods

WHAT DOES IT MEAN TO GO SHOPPING FOR ECO-FOODS? Do you need to become a contemporary forager? Can you never buy another non-organic item? I don't think so. Throughout this book, I will share with you my own experiences and personal reflections from what I have learned. Every day, there is something new to learn about our foods — how they are grown or raised, what the governmental policies are or are not, and how farming affects families all over the world.

The state of our food system can feel daunting; and yet I believe that together we can visit the issues and celebrate the choices we can make for change. Every day a new project emerges from creative people offering up a potential solution to some food-related problem. Our job, as shoppers, is to try to encourage them and buy the fruits of their labor.

How do we know what to buy? We won't know exactly. What was today's best choice may not be tomorrow's. Yet every effort we make is one toward health ... for the Earth and for all of us. What is it like to shop for eco-foods, armed with the bit of knowledge you will get from this book?

Let's start by heading to the local grocery store for one example of shopping for eco-foods. Remember, it will be much different after you become accustomed to making your selections. This rather long excursion is intended to share with you the types of considerations a typical eco-foods shopper might face in a conventional store. Natural-foods stores and other alternatives such as farmers' markets or community-supported farms make eco-foods shopping a lot more fun.

I am not a big fan of grocery shopping, but I do like mastering the food scene for my family. Shopping can scratch a big itch if I feel I have chosen well and waxed poetic with homemade recipes. But it can also leave me feeling sad and frustrated if the choices seem more manufactured than harvested.

We are headed to one of those really big markets. (My sister-in-law uses that term, "I'm going to the market." I like how it sounds.) It is a "super" store stocked with 64,000 products presented in the most researched and attractive way possible.

With my laptop computer nestled into the cart where the children used to sit (were they really that small once upon a time?), the first things I see are processed foods on sale. Cheese crackers, two for $4, or sugar-free cookies, also two for $4. I hate to start out whining, but already we have arrived at a potential source of genetically modified organisms (GMO). In the next chapter, we will do a quick stop at the GMO issue; we will review it more thoroughly in Chapter 10.

> "Natural-foods stores and other alternatives such as farmers' markets or community-supported farms make eco-foods shopping a lot more fun."

About those sugar-free cookies, I can only guess what makes them sugar-free. There it is. Aspartame. Oh wait, what is that on the label? "Excess consumption may have a laxative effect." That would be polydextrose. I will talk more in Chapter 9 about additives and some resources (books and websites) that confirm their safety (or danger).

Next, here on the top shelf, we have a private label, an industry term for items labeled with the store name. It means the packers put together the product specifically for the supermarket or chain. In this case, it is apple juice at only 99¢ for two quarts! I am not surprised at the low cost. US apple-growers are competing with producers in China, particularly in the juice category. Unfortunately, apples are one of the most pesticide-laden crops. Could this juice be made from apples grown locally, using integrated pest management (IPM) or organic practices? There is no indication. Questions about international versus local sources as well as those about production practices are often the

Shopping tip

Questions about international versus local sources as well as those about production practices are often the first ones to ask.

first ones to ask. They are important considerations, so full chapters are devoted to each one.

Here is tuna on sale, with three labels on the can. First is the "Please Recycle" arrow-triangle, reminding me to separate my trash — that I can do. The next says, "Meets American Heart Association food criteria for saturated fat and cholesterol for healthy people over age 2." Then there is the dolphin-safe label. We want to save dolphins from unruly nets. One last check: albacore (the tuna) is in the yellow area of my handy Audubon endangered-fish wallet card, meaning there are some concerns. (The yellow section of the card stands for caution.) In Chapter 12 you will learn a bit more about fish and how to download your own free wallet card. For today, we will forego tuna.

Finally, baked beans are on sale — five for $4 … less than a dollar a can. Doesn't the container cost at least a dollar? And if molasses and garlic and onion and pork bits are all added through a yummy sauce, how much can the growers be getting for their pea beans? We'll talk later about how little the growers get from our grocery tab. In the meantime, let's move on …

> "Wouldn't it be fun if we had an X-ray machine that showed pesticide residue and contaminated water on each fruit? We might choose very differently then."

The Produce Department

On to the veggies section, where a big banner says, "Fresh from the world's best growers." Looking at the rows of brightly colored fruits, it is hard to make the connection with someone's labor or a field somewhere.

First, we have the on-sale produce items. Red and white seedless grapes from Chile are advertised as less than half price at 97¢ per pound. To my right, we have extra large Red Delicious apples for $1.29 a pound — the little label on each fruit gives no state or country of origin. My guess is that they come from Washington State, as they have a distinctive and uniform look about them. Next we have California seedless navel oranges, jumbo-sized and half-price at 49¢ a pound. Well, at least we know where they are from. They, too, seem to have that unusually perfect look. A woman next to me spied a beauty in the back of the bin. We have become extremely discriminatory when it comes to selecting our basket of produce. The perfect-fruit syndrome — we look for the most cosmetically satisfying. Wouldn't it be fun if we had an X-ray machine that showed pesticide residue and contaminated water on each fruit? We might choose very differently then.

Also featured on sale are tangerines from Florida instead of the usual clementines. (Most clementines are grown halfway around the globe, and the nonrenewable resources to get them here are considerable.) Apparently little bugs prevented further imports this season. I can only imagine the financial devastation to those growers.

Out of the sale items and onto the tables. Here are the rest of the apples — now these say Washington — but they don't say how they have been grown. "Excuse me," I say to the store worker, "where are the locally grown apples?" It is January, and due to special three-month storage units, I know local apples should be reappearing from this past season. Fumbling (here comes the store manager), the produce staff pulls out a bag of Empire apples that look great. Uneven coloring and crisp-looking exteriors promise a great-tasting fruit. "How do you know they are from the Northeast?" I ask the produce guy. "They don't say so."

"I just know they're from New York State," he replies. But another man, unpacking bags of celery (also from California), says, "No way — those are from Connecticut, I'm sure." Well, I am glad he's sure. I'm not. How would I know?

"Wait … here are some organic apples," says the manager, knowing how I am and how I can be appeased with an organic version. In a small wicker basket on the side sit a couple of dozen organic apples. Some of them are a little mealy-looking, and one has a particular insect mark I recognize that certainly would not affect me, but compared with the organic apples of the early days, these rival the best of the bunch — maybe because they, too, look as varied as they would on a tree. Many of the apple growers in the Northeast have been using Integrated Pest Management (IPM) practices. For today, I think I will buy the local (New York or Connecticut) and IPM-grown versus the organically grown. Being informed doesn't mean you will feel 100 percent sure of your decisions. Tomorrow, I could choose the organic version.

Here comes George, our produce manager. Now I have the attention of the general manager and the produce manager — we have come to know each other over the years. Michael, the general manager, tries really hard to please his grown-up hippy crowd with Earth-friendly foods. He tells me that the supermarket chain, as one of the worldwide grocery giants, is often despised by the "beyond liberal" residents of this college town. "The company does these surveys of shoppers from the various stores," he explains, "and consistently I have to go to meetings and answer for being hated by the community." He does try. Last summer, Michael invited an organic grower in to set up a little farmer's market in the store and give demonstrations. It was a big success and a real effort at bringing attention to the importance of buying local.

As often happens, Michael and George and I get into a conversation about how hard it is to actually buy from local growers. They work with a growers' cooperative in the area that can be "inconsistent and sometimes just doesn't come through with the product. We just can't be in a position to lose the business," they say. They continue trying to order directly from the grower and avoid the chain's warehouse altogether. It's tricky, but they work at it, knowing their customers really want locally-grown produce. "They want grapes, too," Michael says, acknowledging grapes usually come from other countries. "What do we do about that?" It is an ongoing discussion — one we won't finish today — but a discussion nonetheless, and that's the good news.

Back to produce. Pears. I have such an issue with pears. I don't think I have purchased a ripe pear from a grocery store in years. Again, I don't know where they were grown but I do know they are as hard as rocks. I try putting them in paper bags for a few days, but then they seem to be all bruised by the time they ripen. The labels say, "Ripe when yields to gentle pressure." That's nice, but some parts yield, and other parts feel hard. I guess pears are best off the tree, ready to eat when truly ripe. What to do? Forget the pears!

Here are the bananas. Even though bananas are not local, I know Chiquita has been working with the Rainforest Alliance, one of the many wonderful partnerships toward sustainability you will learn about throughout this book. Oh, dear, no Chiquita brand today. Now, wait, here is a bunch of certified organic bananas. Who says they are organic? How about these little baby bananas? They look perfectly ripe, not too perfect, but no information. Should I hazard it, or decide the origin is too many miles away? "Eat seasonally!" screams in my head. No bananas today.

Peppers! They are so pretty. Yellow, red, orange, purple, and green — how festive! The red peppers are even on sale for $1.99. Do we have to take a closer look? I really want to buy these. The red ones indicate the brand name, and the yellow ones say "produce of Israel." The rest say nothing. They go into the cart, but with the knowledge that they are out of season and from far away.

Perpendicular to the aisles is the cooler, which gets zapped by the little mist spray every 15 minutes or so. The first items are absolutely beautiful — huge organic leeks intermingled with red chard labeled "Organically Grown with Pride and Integrity." (The chard heads into the cart.) Gorgeous dandelion, beet, and turnip greens wrap around anise bulbs and bright purple kale. This is a magnificent presentation of things that may even be grown locally, and some are certainly grown organically. One man stops by this enticing smorgasbord of colorful greens and tells me the broccoli rabe is beautiful today. When I mention the infrequent visitors to that corner of the cooler, he responds, "Americans don't eat greens." Another friend wheels by and suggests no one knows how to cook greens anymore.

Next to the greens, and plenty popular, are the bags of what-were-once-presumably-carrots. It looks like at least a half dozen people have popped a bag of those machine-carved, bred-for-skinniness, orange snack items into their baskets. (Yes, I am guilty. When no carrots are available to me through our community farm, I have been known to get a bag or two to solve the hurry-up-I've-got-to-get-something-in-the-lunch-box dilemma. However, I do prefer to have my carrots a little dirt-stained and with a few roots left on.)

Let's keep moving. Here are the exotics: kiwis (from Greece), blueberries and raspberries (from Chile), and strawberries (from California). Let me remind you it is January.

On to the tomatoes. I like the potential of those little grape tomatoes, but they don't have much flavor. I had great hopes when they first came out that my kids would like them. They will eat the tiny berry-sized versions from the vine when they are in season at the community farm or if we grow them ourselves. But, no such luck, these taste like most other tomatoes these days — flavorless. Here are some vine-ripened tomatoes for 97¢ a pound. They may be good, but at that price, how can the farmer make any money at all?

Truthfully, only one tomato product here looks as if it may have some flavor: organic tomatoes on the vine for $3.99 a pound. Wow, that's a lot of money. If I put back the peppers from Israel, maybe I could make pasta that highlights these luxuries. What??? These organic tomatoes are from Israel, too — no lie! I am not making this up. Something else from halfway around the world and out of season. I give up. The peppers go back, the tomatoes go back, and the local IPM-grown apples and organic red chard are in.

Now, let's not lose faith. Here is a wonderful item: from Waterfield Farm, fresh, hydroponically-grown basil, produced right here in Amherst, Massachusetts. The growers use natural fertilizers from fish raised in a solar system, with no pesticides. They have had their problems, but they continue to work at sustainable systems. I have been to their operation, all under the type of dome you might see covering a sports arena. The idea of growing without soil doesn't sit well with me, but I know that what they are trying to do is innovative and working toward a healthy planet.

The amount of organic in the store is quite respectable, with small quantities of items in most categories, from sweet potatoes to okra, displayed in little wicker baskets. There used to be an organic section, but now each organic item is displayed next to its conventional counterpart. I do like the choice right at my fingertips. This is a sign of progress, one I am grateful for.

> ## Shopping tip
> *I worked with growers in Wisconsin who now grow potatoes under a set of standards awarded the "Protected Harvest" label.*

Potatoes, now that is something near and dear to my heart. Potatoes are 79¢ a pound in the bulk bin. The organic five-pound bag is $2.99, which means they cost 60¢ a pound. I would tell you that is a no-brainer, except I am still sad. I worked with growers in Wisconsin who now grow potatoes under a set of standards awarded the "Protected Harvest" label. These production standards were developed with the World Wildlife Fund and the University of Wisconsin over a very long time and have helped the growers reduce chemicals significantly in that state. The potatoes are called "Healthy Grown," and I would like to buy them to show my support. The problem is, they aren't here. These organic potatoes are from Colorado, so it isn't as if they are more local than Wisconsin. I guess I had better talk to George.

There is a large quantity of organically grown and (apparently) local winter squash, rutabagas, cabbage, and celeriac. If we weren't members of a community farm that supplied these items, they would be destined for the cart. These are the perfect foods — local, in season, and sustainably grown.

Here we are at the soy-products cooler; I am not sure why soy products are in with the produce. I remember coming to this area every week when the children were small: they liked tofu "hot dogs," which became a staple. Once they learned the taste of the real version, I had a hard time convincing them of the merits of the soy version. Lately, my daughter's best friend appears at school with a cold tofu pup in her lunch box, so it has been deemed "cool."

The "health food" section

Let's move on to the separate "health food" section. New Yogi Tea products: chai in boxes. That looks interesting. I like this company and its philosophy. It supports an award breakfast for sustainable businesses at the annual Natural Products Expo. The winners are always great, innovative natural-food businesses that are trying to stay true to their values.

There are some other really good tea companies out there. I try to track which countries the herbs come from and whether they are certified organic. They may not emphasize it on their boxes, so you might want to check their websites before your next shopping trip.

Organic cheese, organic butter, organic milk. Why is one brand of organic milk stuck over here in an out-of-the-way section, while the other is over with the conventional milk? My guess is corporate buy-out. To be safe, I'll put this out-of-the-way one in the cart. I wonder if the same thing goes for the one soy milk over there versus these six or seven different brands here. Look at this: soy milk made with organic soybeans, packed for the store, and inexpensive. Remember, if it is organic, it cannot contain GMOs. I must remember to thank Michael.

> ## Shopping tip
> Remember, if it is organic, it cannot contain GMOs.

Organic cereal, that's good ... no GMOs ... $7.99 — no, thank you. I am sorry, but I have a limit. Price is often pointed to as the reason for not purchasing more sustainable foods. It is true, however, that we in North America pay a distortedly low price for our food in general. If paying more means more for the farmer, I am grateful for the opportunity. Sometimes the price is just too far out of my range. These decisions are not easy. Here is some granola for less, but I love to make my own. Let's just get the organic millet puffs.

> "... we in North America pay a distortedly low price for our food in general. If paying more means more for the farmer, I am grateful for the opportunity."

Snack foods, natural style. No, I think I'll pop my own popcorn from the ears the farm grew this summer. (I remember when a farmer friend first brought us some popcorn on the cob. I didn't know what to do with it. I felt like the urban school child who didn't know milk comes from cows. I finally figured out how to press off the kernels into a pan of oil, but not before I tried popping the whole cob.) Wait, here is my favorite pretzel company with an organic product. I think I'll try it. (That was an impulse buy.)

Organic baby foods. I am no longer in the market, but I do notice they say quite clearly, "No GMO." They may not be able to say that for much longer unless something changes with our GMO labeling laws. Chapter 10 describes more about this challenge. Organic teething cookies — it's such a good thing to have these choices. I hate to admit it, but my attitude about my own health is fairly minimal. I try to stay healthyish. However, when it comes to my children's health, particularly their food consumption, it is an entirely different matter. I am like a she-wolf ready to pounce on anyone adulterating my kids' diets. I have worked very hard to introduce nutritious and yummy foodstuffs since birth. In their early days, I was vehement, and I believe it has paid off.

Out of the "health foods" section and into cheese. How do I know if these have rBGH (a growth hormone given to cows which boosts milk production) or antibiotics in them? I don't. I think I will stick to the small-farm products, the organic versions and some of the European choices for now. Europe has been ahead of the US on some of these issues. Having visited a few cheesemakers in France on a sustainable agriculture tour, I feel the comfort that comes from putting the farmers' faces on foods.

Nuts and raisins. "What happened to my Pavitch organic raisins?" I ask the store worker. "You usually have the six-packs I can send with my kids." He shrugs his shoulders. What about those organic fruit roll-ups? Of course, ever since my daughter traded hers for a commercial version at school, she complains, "Can't we have the real ones?" I then put her through a long explanation of how they aren't the real ones; they are not made with real, 100 percent fruit. After much whining, I threaten to make our own again, and she is quiet. The organic store-bought ones will do.

Coming around the corner, I am met by another source of this family's food fights, packaged, processed lunches. I realize these are a similar solution to the TV dinner of my youth, but I cannot bring myself to buy them. The children will just have to continue to complain. Thank goodness for my daughter's best friend. I remind her, "Remember, Zoe brings tofu pups for lunch!" Oh, yeah, packaging is not that cool.

The fish counter

Here we are at the fish counter. I have my trusty Audubon wallet card on me, so I compare the available fish to the "green, so go ahead" area. Flounder sits in the case. Remember fried flounder sandwiches? Audubon says, "No go." And swordfish? We served swordfish at our wedding many years ago. I wish I had known then what I know now. Swordfish is over-fished and depleted in the Atlantic ocean, although new systems are under way for recovery. But look at that catfish and those mahimahi fillets. They fall in the "go-ahead" zone on the card.

What is really scary is that shrimp — cooked and uncooked — take up almost half the counter. "How much shrimp do you sell?" I ask the counterman. "Depends

Shopping tip

"Shrimp fall in the orange-to-red zone on the card. There are some serious environmental and social concerns about how shrimp are farmed."

on what's on sale, of course," he says, "but usually more than anything else, except maybe salmon. Over the holidays we order a lot more." Shrimp fall in the orange-to-red zone on the card. There are some serious environmental and social concerns about how shrimp are farmed, discussed further in Chapter 12. Don't worry, plenty of other fish get the go-ahead. Ideally, if we take the time today to avoid buying certain species, we will all have a future with oceans of plenty.

Here is the regular coffee section. Unfortunately, I know there is no Fair Trade, shade-grown, or organic coffee over here, unless Michael has been able to add it to his inventory in the past few weeks. The coffee industry is quite a mess for Mother Earth and for many small farmers who live on her. We will talk more about this in Chapter 8. (Stop the presses: Michael has been successful in supplying Fair Trade, organic beans from a local roaster!)

The meat department

In the next chapter, I will introduce you to the use of antibiotics in the raising of meats. Until recently, I would have said this was the biggest frustration I have at our local grocery — no antibiotic-free meat or poultry. Today, I am grateful to say, there are choices. This is very exciting and it made my Christmas dinner. With so many wonderful vegetables from the community farm available in the storage cooler, I had no idea what to serve as the main course and still stay Earth-friendly. Then I spied the free-range, all natural, antibiotic-free, and no-artificial-ingredients chicken breasts, ready to be stuffed and doused with raspberry sauce (frozen from the farm). I ran to thank Michael. Nice job! He brushed me off with an ever-so-small smile.

In addition to the chicken, there is Coleman Natural Beef — no hormones, no antibiotics — and Bramble Hill, our local sheepherder's lamb and sausages. I know these sheep have ample outdoor space to roam. "How are these natural products selling?" I ask the butcher. "Well, we sell them," he replies, "but only about 30 percent of what we get in ... we can't buy less than a case at a time. We lose money on them, but we need to carry them for some people." He continues, "You know they are a better product, certainly. But, it's a price thing. Guess what's been on sale? Products from their conventional factory farm competitors. So what can a big family do when you can get the same thing you might pay $4.99 a pound for here in the natural section for 70¢ a pound down there?" Good question. After explaining that the butchers try all the products when they are first introduced, he said, "To be honest, they have a bit of a gamey taste. I guess it's a lot like tomatoes or eggs, with good, fresh quality items, they taste stronger." I say, you mean they have taste. "Yeah, I guess that's it," he laughs.

Maple syrup … buy local; cereal … make my own (or back to the natural foods section); pasta sauce … make my own from tomatoes and basil from the farm or buy organic; pasta … yes, this is a dilemma. I go for the certified organic version, $1 a box more than the private store label. That's okay with me.

Flour. I like Hodgson Mill whole wheat, with no preservatives, artificial coloring, flavoring, BHA, or BHT. I think I will try their pasta flour. The kids and I can have fun trying this age-old tradition of making noodles. I also choose another flour because it is from a company only two hours up the road. That's a good thing — buy local! Organic flour is not available here. Maybe I should talk to Michael. I wonder what he thinks when he sees me coming, poor guy.

International foods — I will splurge sometimes, but not tonight. Beans — I buy them in bulk at a local health food store. Chips and snacks — stick to the organics, splurge on pretzels. Butter — buy local (another Vermont company "just up the road"). Yeast — I need it for baking bread and pizza dough, so it is a moot point. Sour cream and cream cheese — not organic. I am falling down on the job as we rush along. This really does happen to me. As I start out in produce, I have loads of energy, examining closely, taking extra time. But by the time I hit these aisles, my fortitude is virtually flattened. Then I must remember, buying eco-foods is important, and there is no "perfect" way to do it. With every effort made, it is an action toward change. We can do this … together.

In the yogurt section I see Stoneyfield, and even though I know a huge overseas multinational has bought the company, it is still organic, and the founder grew the company with the Earth in mind. And it is packaged in small tubs for quick lunchboxes, which will appease my children. So my enthusiasm returns, and I know I can leave this place with enough food to feed a family of a four.

Shopping tip

In the yogurt section I see Stoneyfield, and even though I know a huge overseas multinational has bought the company, it is still organic, and the founder grew the company with the Earth in mind.

Then I buy the shredded cheeses. "What's up with that?" you ask. Yes, I make my own salsa and sauce, freeze tomatoes and fruits, bake breads and granolas. And I buy shredded and mixed cheeses. I don't know why, I just do. Remember, progress, not perfection.

Got milk? Yes, I do. Remember, I bought it in the far-off natural foods section. Other local and organic milks are available here, but I'll keep what I have. Another surprise treat: local eggs from the farm where I get my turkey each Thanksgiving. It is nice to support a truly local business. Frozen section — I won't even go down the aisle. Nothing there for me, and the ice cream is just too tempting. Peanut butter — natural, but not organic. Doughnuts, don't I wish. Sandwich bread — 100 percent whole wheat, but not organic. Finding organic grains is very frustrating. I wish we had more access. Here is bread made in Vermont — add it to the cart.

No, I am not stopping for a fresh muffin or baguette — let's head home. As I stand at the checkout counter, I think of the words of Brewster Kneen, an early hero of sustainable agriculture-turned-GMO activist, who suggested individual actions, "such as saying to the checkout clerk in a voice audible to those near you that you would like to buy this canola oil (or whatever), but not if it is genetically engineered or comes from GE crops. Unfortunately", you add, "the product is inadequately labeled and does not provide this essential information."[1]

I never seem to have that much gumption. I just choose eco-foods, one grocery trip at a time, to the best of my ability. Thanks for joining me. Now that you have had a taste of one woman's shopping experience, let's take a tour of the stories behind the eco-foods issues.

2

"GMOs, Pesticides, and Drugs, Oh, My!"

THERE WAS A DAY WHEN A CHAT WITH OUR CORNER GROCER WAS THE NORM. We trusted the local supermarket manager, as we would a pharmacist, to tell us what was in season, what fish or meat had just come in, or what new products were worth trying. The thought that there might be residue from chemicals or antibiotics or even manipulated genes in or on our groceries never crossed our minds. Today, we just aren't so sure.

Pesticides

Pesticides include all the "-icides" used on pests: insecticides on insects, herbicides on weeds, and fungicides on bacteria. Headline, *USA Today*, June 29, 2000: "Report: Common Herbicide likely causes cancer." The Environmental Protection Agency (EPA) upgraded another popular chemical, "the weedkiller of choice for farmers growing corn, sorghum, citrus fruits and other crops," from a possible to a likely carcinogen. The EPA considers 60 percent of all herbicides, 90 percent of all fungicides, and 30 percent of all insecticides carcinogenic: cancer-causing. And the list keeps getting longer. Since pesticides are designed to kill living organisms, it should not be a surprise that they can harm humans. But traditional agriculture has become dependent on them.

How did this all come to pass? The original culprit was malaria, a disease carried from victim to victim by mosquitoes, which are great at giving miniature shots of the disease through their mouthparts. Malaria was and still is one of the most significant killers of our time. In the 20th century, it killed 100–300 million people, mostly infants and young children, and it infects and debilitates hundreds of millions more each year.[1] DDT, an insecticide that killed mosquitoes, was the first serious bug-killer invented to save lives, and it did. Its inventor, Paul Muller, was honored with the Nobel Prize.

> "The EPA considers 60 percent of all herbicides, 90 percent of all fungicides, and 30 percent of all insecticides carcinogenic: cancer-causing."

Since this elixir was so effective against mosquitoes, it was reasoned that it might also be a powerful tool on farms to save crops, or even in summer communities to improve tourism. DDT grew in popularity — its use became overuse. In the early 60s, however, a wise biologist, Rachel Carson, shared research from many scientists on the effects of DDT on life — wild and human — in three *New York Times* articles and later in her book *Silent Spring*. Carson claimed that DDT accumulated through the food chain from algae to birds to humans and was then passed on to our own offspring. As you can imagine, not everyone was happy with the news. Thankfully, many smart people backed her solid research and began a series of changes in policy, resulting in the banning of DDT, at least in the US.

This winter, I learned a bit about an international treaty being worked up to ban persistent organophosphates (POPs), the DDT type of pesticides. It was only in 2001 that some developing countries agreed to no longer use these chemicals. It doesn't sound like much of a story, but it is. In 1981, the Institute for Food and Development Policy published *Circle of Poison: Pesticides and People in a Hungry World*, a book detailing the action of some multinational chemical companies that continued to sell or "dump" large quantities of chemicals overseas because they could. They were legal over there, just not here. US manufacturers exported more than 465 million pounds of pesticides in 1990, while more than 52 million pounds were banned, restricted or unregistered for use in the United States.[2] We won't even begin to discuss the ethics involved. Instead, we will simply look at what happens to the food sprayed with these known killers. We import it … and eat it. This is referred to as "the boomerang effect," and it affects us in a big way. The US imports of fresh vegetables from fiscal year 2001 were valued at $2,476,462,000 and for fresh fruits was valued at $2,025,598,000.[3]

The FDA samples only a small percentage of our imports for residue tests. Even if illegal pesticides are detected, they may still make it to our grocery aisles. One example is from a close examination in 1986, which found that 73 of 164 shipments containing illegal pesticide residues were allowed to reach the marketplace. Of these, in only eight cases were the importers assessed damages.[4] With freer trade policies coming from GATT (General Agreement on Tariffs and Trade) and NAFTA (North American Free Trade Agreement), there may be fewer border inspections.

> "The weeds, bugs, and diseases are winning. We must support and encourage those using IPM (integrated pest management) or organic methods."

How much pesticide is really used in the US these days? With the awareness of its danger and the improvement of the organic market, we might have at least reduced the usage, right? Only slightly! Use of conventional farm pesticides increased from about 400 million pounds in the mid-1960s to nearly 850 million pounds around 1980, primarily because of widespread adoption of herbicides in crop production. Since that time, usage has decreased somewhat, ranging from a low of 658 million pounds in 1987 to a high of 806 million pounds in 1996.[5] The irony is that we are losing the war. Between 1945 and 1989, insecticide use in the US increased tenfold, while crop losses from insect damage almost doubled, from 7 percent to 13 percent.[6] The weeds, bugs, and diseases are winning, but getting off this merry-go-round is no easy task. We must support and encourage those using IPM (integrated pest management) or organic methods. We must support the organizations doing the policy work to stop sales here and overseas of the noxious chemicals.

Thankfully, in August 1996, the US Congress signed the Food Quality Protection Act (FQPA). Certainly there was legislation before, specifically the Federal Insecticide, Fungicide and Rodenticide Act, but it wasn't getting anywhere too fast. The FQPA initiated a long and grueling process of reassessing approximately 9,600 pesticide tolerances and developing new standards for acceptability on future registrations. The Environmental Protection Agency (EPA) has ten years from the signing to accomplish the Act's goals — of which only some are related to the reevaluation. Much of the work has to do with establishing the parameters of "reasonable certainty of no harm," a big change from its previous guidelines, and with deciphering when there is insufficient research to determine a tolerance. In the winter of 2001, Chuck Benbrook and the Consumers Union put together a "Report Card for the EPA" on its implementing of the FQPA (available on the CU website

<www.consumersunion.org>). The EPA is moving at a snail's pace, but one major ban on methyl parathion (a really bad organophosphate) improved its standing. In the meantime, many pro-pesticide campaigners have been working hard on Capitol Hill trying to put their own kibosh on the FQPA.

In the meantime, pesticides exist on our foods. How much, exactly, is tough to figure, but the Environmental Working Group has an amazing website at **<www.ewg.org>** where consumers can check out the contents of a typical grocery cart. The groceries are tabulated and returned with the amount of pesticide they probably contain. In the meantime, it might be helpful to cultivate the habit of washing off all your produce, no matter how it has been grown or where it is from.

Genetically modified organisms

Catchy term, "frankenfoods." The idea of splicing one gene from one thing —could be plant, fish, fowl, or whatever — and putting it into another totally different thing to create a "we-aren't-sure-yet" sounds like it comes right out of the Frankenstein movie, doesn't it? But even though we have altered specific plants, according to a CBS news special aired in 2001, "What Have They Done to Our Food?," the FDA generally considers gene-spliced plants to be the same as the original.

In essence, genes are the instructions contained in the cells of every living thing, telling the organism how to live, breath, reproduce, you name it. For example, one of the genes of Arctic flounder tells it to withstand cold. The idea of genetically "modifying" (or manipulating, however you see it) is that scientists can now take that cold-resistant gene and put it into your favorite strawberry so it will resist frost damage — a real solution for strawberry growers. The problem is, will that strawberry continue to do everything else the way it would have originally? How do we know without years of testing both the berry and our reactions to it?

"We are convinced that the foods that are out there are safe for consumers," says James Maryanski, who oversees biotechnology at the US Food and Drug Administration, the federal agency that polices food safety. He acknowledges that no long-term human health safety tests are required for these foods, "because these are foods that we are real familiar with. These are crops, soy beans, corn, potatoes. We know a lot about those and have a lot of experience with them."[7] It does seem to me if you put a specific gene from one thing that has a quality you want into another thing in order to change it (that is the point after all), then the second thing is changed or different.

Charles Margulis of Greenpeace has stated, "We feel that this is a mass genetic experiment that's going on in our environment and in our diets."[8] We just don't know. That seems to be the mantra around this issue. A variety of surveys indicate consumers want to know if GMOs are in their groceries, but the industry is afraid if we read labels indicating the presence of GMOs, we won't buy them. In Canada in 2001, Loblaw's grocery chain asked organic growers to cover up any GMO-free labeling or "face the prospect of reduced shelf space."[9]

I became rather unnerved when listening to the legendary environmental pioneer Barry Commoner on Earth Day a few years ago at the University of Massachusetts. A wonderful speaker, he explained to us lay folk how scientists have used certain principles to understand DNA structure and the proteins and how they ravel and ignite their applications. The problem with biotechnology, as he could see it, was that some of the scientific principles it relied on were being

> **"... the industry is afraid if we read labels indicating the presence of GMOs, we won't buy them."**

proved wrong. In other words, the rules were changing, so the whole process of modification was resting on loose bedrock. Commoner expressed his concerns about a potential disaster similar to that of the pesticide mess.

Some people are trying to infuse more prudence by applying concepts such as the precautionary principle. According to an article in *Scientific American*, "Although there is no consensus definition of what is termed the precautionary principle, one oft-mentioned statement, from the so-called Wingspread conference in Racine, Wis., in 1998 sums it up: 'When an activity raises threats of harm to human health or the environment, precautionary measures should be taken even if some cause and effect relationships are not fully established scientifically.'"[10] Not everyone is behind this concept.

Have GMOs become established in our food system yet? Yes. Up to 70 percent of processed food in the US market

> **"Up to 70 percent of processed food in the US market contains products of genetic engineering, including soft drinks, catsup, potato chips, cookies, ice cream and corn flakes."**

contains products of genetic engineering, including soft drinks, catsup, potato chips, cookies, ice cream and corn flakes. It is a little like hide-the-GMO-game. They are so ingrained in the food system, we can't even make a choice. This is one of the most serious concerns of GMO opponents. Without knowledge of the gene game, individuals may be exposed to things they may be allergic to. This is why some say we will never see peanuts or other common allergens spliced into anything.

We don't have enough adequate tests. One that did point to the health implications of GMOs was severely questioned. A Bulgarian scientist, Arpad Pusztai, discovered rats fed bioengineered potatoes had thickening of the stomach and intestine linings. His work was published in the respected British journal, *The Lancet*,[11] but he was severely criticized for his findings. Since the controversy, a number of scientists have banded together to reestablish Pusztai's credibility.

The EPA demands that companies carry out a certain number of minimal tests to verify low levels of allergens. Starlink, a genetically modified corn seed product with potential allergen qualities, was refused for human consumption. The EPA did, however, approve it for animal use. So farmers took on the laborious challenge of keeping the corn for humans separated from that for animals. Unfortunately, despite the efforts, Starlink did end up in taco shells and a handful of other products. So Aventis, the multinational that introduced the product, has recalled the product and made compensation agreements with growers to the tune of at least $100 million.

Besides the allergen problem, there are other implications to GMOs, such as environmental and diversity concerns. Since one of the largest investors in biotechnology is also one of the largest investors in pesticides, it may come as no surprise that seeds have been gene spliced to tolerate more pesticide use. Some new varieties of corn have been altered so they will not be killed by certain herbicides, specifically Roundup. This allows growers to spray more Roundup without worrying that it will harm the corn. It kills all the weeds, but not the desired crop.

Another corn manipulation has Bt (*bacillus thuringiensis*), a naturally occurring pesticide, spliced into it. The company that produces this says growers will no longer need to spray pesticides on their crop. Unfortunately, those "survival of the fittest" insects ("superbugs") keep coming back, and once they have learned to stand up to a chemical, it proves ineffective. Bt is one of the few natural pesticides that organic growers are allowed to use. Once these bugs chew through the Bt corn, Bt is going to be useless. So something more significant will no doubt be spliced into the corn, leaving the organic industry with one less available tool.

Unfortunately, many other issues are associated with GMOs. Some of the stories can read like tales of espionage and political intrigue. To expand beyond this momentary stop on the biotech trail, read more in Chapter 10.

Drugs

Now that we've gotten past some of the more commanding areas in the forest of food, what may be lurking next? The overuse of antibiotics has become an established part of raising food animals. When you overcrowd, overstimulate, and overextend the definition of dominion, you are likely to need a miracle cure for the results. Hence, we have overuse of our miracle cures — antibiotics — which are most often meant to kick-start a large weight gain early on or to mend an infection gained from some other stress. This overuse will likely contribute to development of strains of antibiotic-resistant bacteria (just like the superbugs), thus reducing the effectiveness of antibiotics against diseases in humans and animals.

How did this happen, the overuse of something that started out with the intention of saving lives? Using antibiotics on animals began with good intentions. When an animal became sick, the veterinarian prescribed antibiotics, just as for humans. However, antibiotics seemed to help in other ways, helping the animals grow much more quickly, handling the potential instead of the presence of disease. They became the panacea. In the past 15 years, use of antimicrobials for nontherapeutic (non-disease) purposes seems to have risen by about 50 percent.[12] How much is the actual total? Industry and advocates differ. The Union for Concerned Scientists reports, "Our estimates of 24.6 million pounds in animal agriculture and 3 million pounds in human medicine suggests that 8 times more antimicrobials are used for nontherapeutic purposes in the three major livestock sectors than in human medicine."[13]

Again, why do we care? Because those antibiotics are the animal versions of the same ones we use. Cipro, for instance, is the very drug reported as the antidote being administered during the anthrax scares in the fall of 2001. The problem is that these bacteria are building resistance, just as bugs build resistance to pesticides. Hence, the antibiotics aren't working as well on us. Thankfully, we have the option of eating products in which antibiotics have not been used. The Institute of Agriculture and Trade Policy has a great resource, "Eat Well, Eat Antibiotic-Free" on its website **<www.iatp.org>** to help you make and find choices.

Mobilization around this issue is occurring overseas. Both the Centers for Disease Control and the World Health Organization have called for an end to the use of antibiotics as growth promoters in agriculture that we depend on in human medicine. "The European Union has prohibited nontherapeutic agricultural use of antimicrobials that are important in human medicine, such as penicillins, tetracyclines, and streptogramins."[14]

The United States is still behind in making significant changes. With the kind of profits that might be lost by pharmaceutical companies as well as multinational food processors if antibiotics were banned from farm use, a huge battle is surely to ensue. Let's hope it doesn't take a significant epidemic to cut through the line of lobbyists on Capitol Hill.

In the meantime, we can make changes. Every day we can choose antibiotic-free foods or we can support efforts to influence lawmakers on improving humane treatment of animals. We can get involved with campaigns. See the Union of Concerned Scientists website **<www.ucsusa.org>** for a sample letter to the FDA. The good news is, now we know the problem exists. Chapter 11 provides more details on the use of subtherapeutic antibiotics in our meat animals.

Shopping tip

"Every day we can choose antibiotic-free foods or we can support efforts to influence lawmakers on improving humane treatment of animals. We can get involved with campaigns."

3

The Earth First

Were man to perish tomorrow, vines would destroy his mighty temples and grass would soon grow in the main streets of the world. In contrast, the disappearance of plants would be accompanied by the disappearance of man along with every other animal.

— JULES JANICK

WHETHER FRUITS, VEGETABLES, GRAINS, DAIRY, OR MEAT, what we eat starts in the earth. Plants are the key to our survival. Not only do they supply us with our food, they provide us with the air we breathe.

Most of us have little awareness of what it takes to grow a "crop." Words like monoculture, disk row harrow, nematodes, or no-tillage are usually left to those who farm. And yet, it is helpful to start with a basic understanding of what it takes to grow the food we eat and the myriad of issues facing growers.

Agronomy: And how does your garden grow?

To some, how to grow a plant may be old hat, but when I first started in this field, I had no idea. After years of agriculture classes, I am now often heard mumbling the photosynthesis chemical reaction in my sleep. A lot goes into plant production and everything seems to matter, from the weather to the neighbors.

A breeze through botany is in order, starting with plant parts and what they do. The plant consists of all sorts of parts, each one with important functions. If we start at the bottom and work up, the roots are our first focus. Not only does the root anchor the plant in place, it is where plants consume or store a majority of their food and drink, at least in terms of nutrients and water. Its job is to probe the dirt for goodies. Just imagine the root as doing the shopping, unloading, storing, and cooking of the majority of the meals — sounds familiar.

Whether a plant has a taproot system — one big, long root — or a fibrous system with lots of smaller, shallow roots, little root hairs exist and do a majority of the absorbing of nutrients. Think of a fresh carrot before it has been processed for a package: it has little root hairs all over it. Some roots have more hairs than we would guess. For example, a rye plant can have more than 14 billion root hairs that have a total surface area about as large as a football field.[1] The more hairs, the more area to absorb, the more "eating" that plant can do.

The stem is the part of a plant that most often sticks up above ground. Of course, there are exceptions to every rule. Some stems shoot along the ground, like those for strawberries. Some stems are the actual food we eat, such as potatoes and asparagus.

The stem houses the two-lane circular highway for phloem and xylem — that's the up-and-down transport system that delivers food to the plant's leaves, flowers, fruit, and seed. Think of maple syrup. The sap has been stored through the winter and is in the process of thawing and heading to the highway. Tapping the syrup is similar to creating a detour.

Next are the nodes where the buds for branches and leaves attach. The leaves are busy. They may not be doing the lion's share of food prep like the roots, but they are doing some. They absorb sunlight and carbon dioxide, have little holes (stomates) for the most part on the undersides, that regulate how much water and CO_2 goes in and out ... interesting ability.

In the leaves the "chemical reaction-photosynthesis thing" kicks in. One of the things I love about photosynthesis is that humans have not been able to reproduce it. Only plants seem to be able to take a combination of sunlight, carbon dioxide and water and turn it into food and oxygen. And we are awfully lucky they can do this, for without photosynthesis, we would have neither food to eat nor air to breathe. This is the time for applause for the plants. You could always simply say thank you, even to your lawn. Some people believe plants can hear us.

Continuing up the plant elevator to the penthouse is my favorite, the apical meristem. It is where, in most plants, it's all happening. The cells are having a party — dividing and multiplying — to keep the plant growing.

The primary function of plants' more aesthetic parts is to reproduce. The flowers, fruit, and seeds are all working toward procreation. It makes sense. Flowers are beautiful, to attract the pollinators, usually bees and other fly-by-nights that carry pollen grains to another flower's stigma for germination. As in humans, the sperm is delivered to an ovary to meet an egg where the fruit grows. Inside the fruit is the seed(s) that will ultimately start the whole ball rolling again.

Also like humans, plants have a genetic makeup, so when the sperm meets the egg, genes are combined and new seeds with new gene makeups are formed. Experimenting with this interaction is how Gregor Mendel (1822–1884) began his work with peas, and the practice of crossbreeding was born. Combining different pea varieties to produce altogether new pea varieties began a whole new world of investigation. And now we have biotechnology, where combining varieties has been left in the dust. Today scientists have started down an all-new track with gene splicing and manipulation.

> "A more immediate reason to understand a plant's complexity is to begin to build empathy for those who grow our food: farmers."

We know what the plant looks like, how it gets its nutrients and how it reproduces. But there is certainly more to it, of course. Plants have hormones, causing certain growth habits such as reaching for the sun, ripening, or going dormant over the winter. One of the things I love so much about plants is that they are almost as complicated in their functioning as humans. They have self-defense mechanisms against diseases and bugs. They adapt to stressful environments. They respond and go on living.

Why should we as consumers be concerned about the intricacies of plant life? In part because it is high time we began a renewed relationship with what we eat. Understanding a partner in any relationship is critical. A more immediate reason to understand a plant's complexity is to begin to build empathy for those who grow our food: farmers. What we have just learned is only a tiny part of what a grower must understand to produce our next meal.

Soils: It starts with the dirt

Plants stand in the dirt, eat dirt, spread their roots in dirt, drink from the dirt and can get sick from the dirt. So dirt is important … and what we add to it and how we dig in it affects our food. The study of soils involves chemistry, and without going too far into it, let's attempt enough of an overview to be able to understand some issues.

First, "dirt" is slang for the more beloved term, "soil." As a friend says, "It is high time we stopped treating our plants like dirt." Hence, let that dust in the ground be heretofore known as soil. This is an important distinction, because our attitude toward it has and will continue to determine our desire to conserve it. As Fred Kirschenmann, director of the Leopold Center for Sustainable Agriculture writes:

> Not too long ago, soil scientists had reduced soil to "a medium that holds a plant in place" while we artificially feed the plant and control its pests. During this era of soil science, soil was considered "fertile" so long as it contained adequate amounts of macronutrients — nitrogen, phosphorous and potash. Later soil scientists began to recognize the importance of micronutrients — sulphur, zinc, etc. Still later they marked the importance of soil structure and its relation to compaction and erosion. Still later, the importance of earthworms began to be recognized. Still later the importance of the "rate of organic matter turnover" was recognized. Now, in recent months, soil scientists everywhere are beginning to talk about "soil quality" and "soil health." This progression is a progression of "seeing" soil — of seeing it as more than dirt. Now scientists are ready to become lovers of the soil — to know it intimately, to care about it. It is this "inner" seeing that helps us to understand the soil as more than a "medium."[2]

I saw this intensity once, between farmer and his soil, when I visited with Amish farmers in Holmes County, Ohio. Although I did not truly understand what constitutes a rich thriving soil, there was no question that this dark brown fluff they shared with pride and passion was formed through years of work, the kind of daily "showing up," baring and sharing toil and soul, that happens only in multi-decade marriages.

Why is soil worth such devotion? From a farmer's view, it provides the substance of life for the crops. Soil brings plants water, nutrients, and oxygen. It is made up of approximately half mineral and organic particles and half pore space for air and water.

The first half — mineral and organic material — is important because it determines how much nutrition can be passed on to the plant and how much pore space will be available to get it there. Soil is made up of a mixture of gravel, sand, silt, and clay. Getting the right combination of these will make or break the plants' ability to move around, let alone breathe. Think of those red clay soils, particularly in the south, that are heavy and dense, the kind Native Americans used to make pottery. It's tough for a plant to push little root hairs though something so rock-hard solid, which is why the preferable soil for plant growth has a balance of gravel or sand.

Clay is also susceptible to "soil compaction." Think of art class, when the teacher made you squish all the little holes out of the clay before making your prized coil pot. An extensive air-duct system exists in the soil, constructed magnificently by earthworms, nematodes (microscopic worms), and the virtual blockparty teeming underground. Like the hole in the playclay, the soil's airspace can be suddenly shut down by pressure from tractors and other heavy things at ground level, especially if the soil is wet and has a high proportion of clay.

Tractors have long been an issue. How do you plow (or till) the soil (meaning, break it up so seeds have the necessary space to begin germination) and, at the same time, not squeeze all the holes together with the weight of the machine? This is tricky and consequently the subject of several opinions about the best method — some advocate not tilling at all, and others suggest a combination of management practices, such as not working the soil when it is wet.

Getting the right mixture of mineral and organic matter matters not only for the soil's tilth — the physical structure — but also for its ability to provide nutrients to the plants. Foregoing an explanation of "cation exchange capacity," suffice it to say that clay and organic matter both act like magnets to the nutrients plants need. Although clay may not be great for soil compaction, it is great for holding water and gathering nutrients. Plants need 16 major and several other minor nutrients for a balanced diet. Their most favorite meal consists of a combination of nitrogen, phosphorus, and potassium. That's why most bags of fertilizers at garden centers indicate quantity of NPK (the chemical symbols for the above nutrients.) Without soils, the fertilizer we add would simply wash away. But those millions of soil particles grab the nutrients and hold onto them until the plant is ready for them. Thank you, soil.

The only problem is that when we humans assist by adding to the soil certain fertilizers that might contain metals that aren't so good for plants or us — metals such as cadmium, copper, nickel, or lead — the soil holds on to them and subsequently passes them on to the plants. This is why some people have fought the use of sewage sludge on fields. They believe sludge may contain too many metals that might contaminate our food. It also may contain pollutants, bacteria, and other toxic compounds that, if not picked up by plants, get washed away into our groundwater.

We still aren't finished with the soil's miraculous magnetic capability. The combination of minerals and organic matter determines a soil's ability to hold water. Just as soil particles collect nutrients, so do they attract water molecules. Scientists refer to this as "water-holding capacity." Sand is not so good at holding water. Watch flowers in a sandy soil start drooping fairly quickly in a drought, while flowers in soils with high organic matter and clays tend to hang in there a lot longer. When water runs into the groundwater too quickly, it can take along lots of nutrients the soil did not get a chance to attract, such as nitrogen. Just as we don't want toxic compounds in our groundwater, aka drinking water, we don't want too many of the good minerals going there, either. Consider nitrogen, for example. Plants need a healthy portion of this mineral for growth, but Mother Nature does not always wait until the plant has absorbed what it needs before providing the earth with a little shower. The rain can cause any excess nitrogen to drain through the soil pores, past the particles' magnets, and into the groundwater, which is ultimately not good for us.

Pathology: Plants can get sick, too

Plants need doctors for diseases just like we do, although we are a bit more complicated. Growers rely on pathologists, like doctors, to keep them informed, and on chemical companies, like pharmacies, to supply them with medications. The problem is that sometimes when we eat the plants, we end up eating those medications. Like those working in the alternative medicine field, many growers are working on prevention through good nutrition and health maintenance. Let's not go through medical school for plants, but at least understand enough to appreciate the big issues.

A standard introduction into the world of plant pathology is the example of the Irish potato famine. The results of the 1845 disaster were a million Irish dead. Another million and a half escaped, mostly to the US and Canada, all because of a fungus that tore through field after field of potatoes. The poor in Ireland were extremely dependent on this one source of nutrition. (Working with Wisconsin potatoes growers for a winter, I came to learn how packed with nutritional power potatoes really are, full of protein, carbohydrates, potassium, and vitamin C.)

Most people think potatoes came from Ireland, but the truth is that they originated in South America and were brought to Europe around 1570. Unfortunately, the extensive range of varieties did not transfer, so most of the potatoes were the same type. (This is Clue No. 1 to the disaster.) Potatoes are grown from large pieces of seed potatoes; thus, those that went to Europe were large and full of opportunity to house pathogens (Clue No. 2). During six weeks of infestation, the weather was cold and damp (Clue No. 3). These three clues happen to fit nicely with what scientists refer to as the "disease triangle, the three factors necessary for a plant disease: a susceptible plant, a pathogen capable of causing disease in the plant, and environmental conditions favorable for disease development."[3]

The susceptible plant (Clue No. 1) was a vulnerable target for a number of reasons. It had traveled from its native warm environment to an area with cold. Another risk factor — no diversity. Every plant was uniform, so the pathogen could zip through a field in an instant. In its homeland, this potato was raised next door to a different type of potato. When a disease came along, it did not spread at epidemic proportions. This is where the issue of monocultures comes in. The way we farm today is to plant row after row of the exact same type of plant. This sounds fine until a disease or insect comes along. If one plant is susceptible, the entire field is susceptible. If you invest a couple of dollars in a half dozen basil seedlings to make a little pesto, you probably aren't worried about disease. If you invest tens of thousands of dollars into fields of basil to sell off to feed your family for the year, you think very seriously about using any combat tool you can.

> "The way we farm today is to plant row after row of the exact same type of plant. This sounds fine until a disease or insect comes along. If one plant is susceptible, the entire field is susceptible."

Back to the disease path and Clue No. 2. As mentioned, potatoes have more room to house pathogens than tiny seeds do, so the infected boatload could carry plenty of the pathogen that caused late blight. Another scary thing about this particular disease is its ability to spread and ruin stored potatoes practically overnight. Late blight in a one-foot-square section of a storage unit the size of a football field could ruin the entire crop. Recently, at least one of the big manufacturers of potato products put the burden of storage on the grower. No longer will some manufacturers store potatoes on their end; they pass the job on to the growers, just in case.

Finally, to Clue No. 3, the contribution of environmental conditions. Chilly and wet conditions for more than six weeks gave the pathogen its favorite setting. Not all diseases favor cold and wet, but many do. One of the most common management techniques is to avoid working in fields in that type of weather as this aids the spread of disease. Again, this sounds pretty easy, but if a buyer wants potatoes at a specified time and it's been raining for days, the grower is stuck.

Back to the disease path. Many different pathogens attack our plant life — in general, fungi, bacteria, viruses, and nematodes (although the last — microscopic worms in the soil — don't seem to go along with the other three). Fungi have their own kingdom (Animals, Plants, Fungi ...), so you know they must have some clout. They either eat dead plants or they act as parasites on living plants. The names of some these fungi and spores are great — how about oomycetes, smut fungi, zoosporangia or slime molds? Fungi tend to ruin the fruits, not the plants themselves — bad enough if you have acres of orchard to pay your annual salary. Orchardist and grape grower Victor Hanson, in his book *The Land Was Everything: Letter from an American Farmer*, describes fungi as follows: "But may I be brief in their description, for they are foul, yet petty, things that ultimately ooze and drip? Despite all their rank and fetid accomplishment, fruit fungi do not even kill the host, but rather rot and discolor the produce alone. They are sloppy and they stink. The harvest of 'the vinegar vine' is what the Greeks said such grapes become."[4]

Hanson's lack of respect for fungi seems to arise from comparison with bacteria and viruses, which evoke a level of reverence someone might give to a greatest foe. Not to say that these two don't do similar damage. They can ruin just the final fruit, but they can also bore into the deepest regions of a plant, such as the phloem, resulting in black, charred branches or stems, or disfigured leaves. Hanson continues as he describes his true enemy: "What else is it but a tragedy to see the best of a Santa Rose plum orchard ruined in its prime by bacterial gummosis, limbs scorched, tiny plums mummified, the entire enterprise of cultivated trees itself a ruin? In 1979 our small, beautiful plum orchard was charred in the space of a few weeks as the contagion took hold. A beautiful white blossom in the February orchard, deep green young leaves in the March breeze, a good April plum set — and then death by June as leaves and undeveloped plums littered the ground."[5]

As with humans, antibiotics work on bacteria; nothing works on viruses. Naturally, these pathogens build resistance to our attacks, ensuring our continuous scurry to find new drugs. What else do we do? We focus on avoidance, exclusion, and eradication. We work on disease-resistant varieties, and we succumb to pesticides. We study the other options, such as biological control, or improving nutrition, and reducing pollution or carrier populations, such as aphids or gnats. We don't have answers yet. It is as simple as that. Here we are with an understanding of one type of enemy, the disease. Of course, it doesn't end there. On to the weeds!

Weeding out the weeds

What are weeds? Some people refer to them simply as "plants out of place." They are not supposed to be there — uninvited guests, party crashers. Some are considered "noxious." Today weed scientists have added to the definition, "plants that are competitive, persistent and pernicious. They interfere with human activities and as a result are undesirable."[6]

The adjectives do give us a place to start. Weeds are considered competitive. They steal the very sustenance — light, water, and nutrients — from crop plants, and they are usually very good at it. Weeds have an uncanny ability to "get the goods" more often than the featured plant. This depends in part on when the weeds show up and how many descend on the scene. If they get there at the same time as our favored plant and can establish a foothold, they have a distinct competitive advantage. Keeping weeds out until the plant is well established is key. Even if they are kept out early on, weeds tend to grow very quickly and can catch up before you know it. The ultimate disgrace occurs when some weeds exude toxins into the soil that actually prevent other plants from growing. This is known as allelopathy.

Weeds are also persistent. As any home gardener knows, a weed removed one day surely means another will take its place the next. How do they keep coming back? The seeds are the culprits — too many for too long! Weeds produce thousands of tiny travelers, seeds built for dispersal with little hooks, feathers, or other physical adaptations to make hitching a ride via wind, rain, lint, or anything else that passes by — including the family dog — an easy trip. They also wear extremely trusty armor and have the ability to sleep (dormancy) until it is their turn to move into action.

Finally, weeds are pernicious, which means they can be more than just a serious pain in the neck. They can cause tremendous loss of crops and soil use. Like any plant, weeds have different lifestyles. Some are annual (they come and go in one growing season), others are biennial (they return in their second year, to produce seeds), and others are perennial (they keep coming back year after year after year).

As you can imagine, the war is on between grower and weed, and what do you think is the farmer's number one ammunition? Pesticides — actually herbicides in this case. Many growers certainly try hoeing and other forms of mechanical control. They try mulches that keep the weeds down and contribute to soil retention. They try crop rotation: moving the plantings to different places each year.

How do farmers kill just the weeds and not the crop plants, you ask? Good question. Monsanto has introduced a new genetically modified corn built to resist the favorite herbicide of many farmers: Roundup. "Roundup-ready" corn can take all the herbicide a farmer can spray and still be standing. That means there may be more pesticide residue than if the grower had to be more specific in the application.

Entomology: Bugs, bugs and more bugs

Now it is time to pull out the microscopes and examine the biggest competitor of all: the bug. Bugs have been around a lot longer than we have, and for good reason — they have been working at it. As described in an entomology textbook, "Insects have lived on the earth for about 350 million years — compared with less than 2 million for man — and during this time they have evolved in many directions to become adapted to life in almost every type of habitat and have developed many unusual, picturesque and even amazing features."[7]

These critters are tricky. They tolerate and adjust. They beat us at our own game. They want what we want ... to live. And we all want to use food to do so. But we also need bugs. About one-third of the world's crops depend on insects for pollination. We need certain insects to ensure the growth of food, and yet we also know insects are responsible for a great deal of damage. According to the Smithsonian entomology website, **<www.entomology.si.edu>** "As pests and human competitors they destroy or eat $5 billion; as disease vectors, insects weaken or kill 200 million people per year."[8] In addition to feeding on the same food we do, they are great at carrying disease and passing it on to unknowing victims. Malaria, black plague, and any number of epidemics have been transmitted by our little friends/foes.

WEBSITE

Insects have very interesting and complex lives, with different stages from larvae to adult. Their systems vary and their palates change accordingly. Some have mouthparts that act like sponges; others can actually pick up a person's skin, cut it with a sword-like appendage, then lap up the blood (a great fun fact that will engage a child in the world of bugs). Insects' behavior is as varied as the number of species — and there are literally thousands of different types of bugs in an average backyard!

Entomologists can spend a lifetime understanding just a few of these bugs. Farmers have considerably less time to understand their potential enemies. For many years, farmers were instructed to follow a schedule, a seasonal

Shopping tip

"We get to set our own standards, deciding how much damage we will tolerate on our fruits and vegetables, versus accepting chemical sprays on our food. Remember, we send a message every time we buy."

Keep those pear thrips out of the maple syrup

Even maple syrup can suffer from little pesky bugs ... and I do mean little. Years ago, I worked for entomologist Craig Hollingsworth on his crusade to keep our sap running. Actually, the Massachusetts Maple Growers Association had asked the University of Massachusetts to study the behavior of pear thrips – a nasty leafeater that had done a number on Vermont in 1988 and threatened to decimate the trees of our state.

To this end, researchers studied the thrips' behavior through a variety of means. My assignment was to track their presence, using yellow sticky pads, at a handful of maple operations at various times of the day. Pear thrips show up in early spring, having overwintered in the soil, to feed on swollen buds and newly expanding leaves. By placing yellow pads coated with a sticky substance at ground level and at intervals of 5–15 feet up the tree, one can capture a sample of the insect several times a day and track the population.

This sounds all very simple and important, but there are a few potential glitches: the thrips are less than 2 mm in size; their most notable characteristic, besides feathery wings, is a thumb-like appendage on the left side (this creature is about the size of a crumb – looking for a such a tiny body part is tricky, to say the least); and tracking their behavior means a lot of waiting. Needless to say, I failed "scientific dedication" when I skipped a last reading one Friday afternoon due to improper clothing selection that morning – shorts and black flies don't mix.

The truth is, this very dedication is what saves our maple syrup from unnecessary pesticides. My days as a scientist never really took off. However, that day my empathy and gratitude did. Thank you to the entomologists who take the time to understand the minutiae in the fields, groves, and orchards. Without them, these tiny pests could destroy a whole lot of our food supply.

calendar of spraying to rid the orchard or field of what might be serious damage. Today many farmers don't follow the calendar. Instead they follow integrated pest management practices (IPM) or organic procedures and try to understand their foes. They also assess how much damage can be tolerated before a necessary strike. This is referred to as the "economic threshold." How much can we let insects get away with before the damage will seriously affect the crop financially?

This is where we, as consumers, have a role. We get to set our own standards, deciding how much damage we will tolerate on our fruits and vegetables, versus accepting chemical sprays on our food. Remember, we send a message every time we buy. Dr. Lyle Craker, a plant and soil sciences professor at the University of Massachusetts, shares the rule of thumb he grew up with: "For every dozen ears of corn you buy, there should be one ear with a corn worm … that signals the right amount of spray was used." No one likes to find worms in the corn, but if it means less pesticide, I can take the extra minute to break off the wormy tip. Some damage is more acceptable than others. In the early days of organic apples, the fruit was sometimes full of half-moon crescent marks or little black spots, and rather disfigured, all common damage done by apple orchard pests. Today the organic versions look better. We are still lulled, by the many bags of heavily sprayed and waxed apples, into believing that perfect fruit is better. Interestingly, the more perfect it looks, the less likely it really is.

> ### Shopping tip
>
> *"We are still lulled, by the many bags of heavily sprayed and waxed apples, into believing that perfect fruit is better. Interestingly, the more perfect it looks, the less likely it really is."*

Growers try to anticipate what the market (that's us) will bear and follow control systems that will result in our preferences. All sorts of mechanical practices are put into action — mowing and removing winter homes for insect larvae, hanging sticky monitoring tools to track economic threshold, adding oils to cornsilk at designated times, or placing pheromone traps (insect sex attractants) in fields. This fight has been going on for a long time. And chemicals just don't work for us, or on the bugs, which simply build resistance and come back for attack. So we use even more toxic chemicals, and they mutate all over again. Who are we hurting? As in any fight, everyone seems to lose.

Remember, there are more and more growers who are the conscientious objectors, particularly those using IPM and organic methods. The price may be higher for these foods because they can cost the farmer more to produce. Sometimes the price is considerably higher. But this is our opportunity to contribute. By purchasing these foods, we endorse and encourage the change, one shopping trip at a time.

4

How We Got Here from There

OUR TRANSITION FROM HUNTERS/GATHERERS TO FARMERS gave Laura Ingalls Wilder's family a dependable food supply. But as more people populated the West as well as the East, the pressure was on to grow more and more, with some ramifications. The first signs of our overuse appeared during the Dust Bowl, as winds blowing through the Midwest states sucked up our prized soil. We hadn't conserved our soil well enough to keep it on the ground. Next came the Green Revolution, our answer to feeding the world. And today, big agribusiness has taken over the growth of most of our foodstuffs, while family farms disappear from the landscape.

The Dust Bowl blew us away: Lesson No. 1 in overuse

Much of the vast US Midwest was known for its ideal land, perfect for growing abundant crops. But by the mid-1930s, years of deep plowing and planting over and over again, combined with years of drought, caused the Plains winds to raise the dirt into billows of dust. Millions of acres of farmland became useless, and hundreds of thousands of people were forced to leave their homes. This first modern version of overuse provided a painful lesson in caring for our soil — otherwise it might, literally, blow away.

In the early 30s, the panhandles of Oklahoma and Texas had been labeled by *Nation's Business* magazine as the most prosperous region in the United States.[1] Compared with the East, where long lines at soup kitchens were evidence of the Great Depression, the Midwest was booming from great success in the fields. According to the PBS special, "Surviving the Dust Bowl," "The land was green and lush, and the soil so rich, an observer noted, that it looked like chocolate where the plow turned the sod."[2]

Yet that was exactly where the trouble began — turning sod. For the previous 20 years or so, farmers had been breaking millions of acres of earth to plant wheat. It was the gold rush of the Midwest, with "suitcase" farmers (visiting folk who had other jobs and took to farming simply to take advantage of the boom) tilling the soil with heavy tractors. Where a team of horses could plow three acres in a day, the tractor could turn 50. No longer were they working a day, either; these tractors moved through the fields 24/7/365. This wasn't being done by the farm families who had been on the land for years, it was by visitors looking for an opportunity. The book *Americans View Their Dust Bowl Experience* describes it: "Down in the Texas Panhandle the movie mogul Hickman Price set about to show plainsmen what modern commercial farming could really do, how it could apply the large-scale business methods of Henry Ford to the mass production of wheat. His factory farm stretched over 54 square miles and required 25 combines at harvest time."[3]

One "survivor" put it this way: "It produced good. It looked liked the greatest thing would never end. So they abused the land. They abused it somethin' terrible. They raped it. They got everything they could."[4] It became known as the Great Plow-Up. During that time, farmers tore up the vegetation on 5,260,000 acres in the southern Plains, an area nearly seven times the size of Rhode Island.[5]

"When the black blizzards began to roll across the region in 1935, one-third of the Dust Bowl region — 33 million acres — lay naked, ungrassed, and vulnerable to the winds."[6] During the mid 30s, three large storms and plenty of smaller ones swirled the chocolate sod through the air, into people's homes and soup bowls, and it settled as grit between their teeth. In the spring of 1935, a journalist from Great Bend, Kansas, reported that "Lady Godiva could ride through the streets without even the horse seeing her."[7]

It wasn't the constant wheat plantings or extensive tilling that really caused the problem, it was those very things in combination with the drought. Is it true that we would still have that topsoil today had "stewardship" been a part of farming before the rain stopped and the winds began? Most experts believe so. Certainly the tables began to turn when conservation systems began.

Thank goodness for the heroes like Hugh Bennett, an agricultural pioneer trying to instill sound management practices, who took his gospel to Washington, DC, and, working with Mother Nature, created a stir over the dusty winds. Serendipitously, at the same time Bennett addressed lawmakers on Capitol Hill, the East experienced its first storm like those that had occurred in the Plains. Thanks to that first-hand knowledge, the federal government agreed to aggressively support soil conservation in the Dust Bowl.

Two weeks after the worst storm of all — "Black Sunday" — Congress declared soil erosion a "national menace," and the Soil Conservation Service was born. Immediately, training and incentive programs began for strip cropping, terracing, crop rotation, contour plowing, and cover cropping, all to improve soil retention. The rains still did not come, but the "conservation practices reduced the amount of blowing soil by 65 percent."[8] By the end of the 1930s, with far fewer farmers in place, the drought finally ended, and hearty harvests began anew.

Was Mother Nature, angered by the relentless scratches to her soil skin, responsible for the devastation? As scientists tried to give a definitive answer, an opportunity presented itself in 1977 with one of the worst dust storms in history. Meteorologist Edwin Kessler demonstrated with aerial cameras that the dust was coming from West Texas farms that had been plowed and planted, while neighboring New Mexico lands left in grass remained stable.[9]

> "In the early 1960s, new wheat and rice varieties were developed to produce more food per acre. But these varieties responded only to intensive use of chemical fertilizers, pesticides, and irrigation."

How green was the Green Revolution?
Lesson No. 2 in overuse

The next history lesson comes from the Green Revolution, known as a "breakthrough" in scientific discovery. Increased yields as a result of progressive plant breeding meant hope for the end of hunger. Lester Brown of the WorldWatch Institute and others were predicting worldwide famine as population increases showed signs of outstripping potential food sources. In the early 1960s, new wheat and rice varieties were developed to produce more food per acre. But these varieties responded only to intensive use of chemical fertilizers, pesticides, and irrigation. As you can imagine, some of the revolution's results were less welcome than the new miracle yields.

The father of the Green Revolution, Norman Borlaug, won the 1970 Nobel Peace Prize for his contribution to ending hunger. In the 1940s, just as the Dust Bowl settled, Borlaug became the director of a Rockefeller Foundation-funded wheat program in Mexico to help poor farmers. While he was there, he developed high-yielding varieties (HYVs) of wheat. These varieties, combined with a "technological package" — irrigation, chemical fertilizers, and pesticides — were transferred to the subsistence farming regions of the world to stop hunger.

The new system provided increased foodstuffs to indigenous cultures of the Third World with a caveat. Subsistence with these new varieties was not possible without investment in technological "inputs." It was a trade-off. Was it successful? The statistics are conflicting. In a 1997 pro-Green Revolution article in *Atlantic Monthly*, the numbers reflected a significant reduction in starvation. The article reported, "By 1974 India was self-sufficient in the production of all cereals. Pakistan progressed from harvesting 3.4 million tons of wheat annually when Borlaug arrived to around 18 million today, India from 11 million tons to 60 million."[10] It is true that yields increased. Unfortunately, this paints only half the picture.

Vaclav Smil, in his book, *Feeding the World*, describes the results of the introduction of high-yielding varieties and their necessary technologies in terms of both good news and bad: "Their introduction began a profound transformation of traditional agricultures, a worldwide conversion from extensive to intensive cropping. Since 1900 the world's cultivated area increased by only about one-third, but because of more than a fourfold increase of average yields the total crop harvest rose almost sixfold. This gain has been due largely to a more than eightyfold increase of external energy inputs, mostly fossil fuels, to crop cultivation ... This shift from subsistence farming powered by animate energies to agriculture critically dependent on large inflows of fossil fuels has brought a surfeit of food too rich in lipids in affluent countries, and, on the average, adequate per capita supply of basic nutrients in all but a few war-ravaged poor nations."[11]

Those who argue for Green Revolution farming practices point to the decrease in hunger. The downside of this is that, although more food is being produced, access to that food is still the inherent problem. It comes down to the poor's inability to pay for this ever more expensive food. In the subsistence days, poor farmers could grow their own foodstuffs. As Indian scientist Vandana Shiva puts it, "As peasants have become more and more dependent on 'off-farm' inputs, so they have become increasingly dependent on those companies that control the inputs."[12] Ultimately, fewer peasants can farm because they cannot afford the costly chemical fertilizers, pesticides, irrigation, and controlled seeds.

The global growing picture

Third World nations were not the only ones to adopt Green Revolution technologies. North American farmers have also been investing in these methods. The dependence syndrome Shiva refers to has manifested in a slightly different way in developed countries. Our current serf system has different players — the "lords" are the transnational corporations, while the "peasants" are the families who keep hanging on to what they can.

The type of subsistence farming we think of in developing countries began to slide away here in North America during the beginning of the industrial revolution and continued as farm families began working in factories to supplement incomes in order to buy the new inventions we were all clamoring for, from washers and dryers to television sets.

In the US at the beginning of the century, 5,739,657 farms each worked an average of 147 acres; 39.2 percent of the population lived on their farms. Today, less than 2 percent of the US population lives on the farm. The average farm today is 487 acres. The number of farms lost from the beginning to the end of the century? 3, 827,798.[13]

What happened to them all? As is happening overseas, the small farmer in the US cannot afford the inputs necessary to grow modern hybrid varieties. Not only must farmers continue to invest in the big three (fertilizers, pesticides, and, in some places, water), they also grow in monocultures (one crop/one field), which calls for big equipment. "Whereas food prices (at the consumer level) have long been stagnant because of overproduction, costs of manufactured inputs have soared. Farmers have been driven into debt to cover the costs of $40,000 tractors and $100,000 harvesters, and by and large their slim profit margins have not been enough to cover debt service, thus leading to waves of bankruptcies and foreclosures."[14]

The few farmers left do not resemble the agrarian lifestyle we like to recollect from our childhoods. The majority of the food being grown for our plates comes from agribusinesses or multifamily operations. As intensive growing methods took over, farm families saw that the only solution to their problem was economy of scale. If they were to compete with the guy down the street, they had to have that many more acres and be able to promise that much

> "The few farmers left do not resemble the agrarian lifestyle we like to recollect from our childhoods. The majority of the food being grown for our plates comes from agribusinesses or multifamily operations."

more quality product at the cheapest price. So if they decided to stay in farming, the big buyout had to begin.

With fewer growers in general, the pressure on supply companies to stick with intensive inputs has become even greater. The sales force behind the inputs has been ever more aggressive, suggesting to farmers that reducing chemicals or, even more drastically, adopting organic methods, would be an impossible risk. "Big money is at stake in maintaining the capital-intensive nature of modern farming, which makes countries and farmers dependent on suppliers of inputs. Clearly, immense profits would be lost if a move to alternatives and indigenous paths were to lead to lowered dependence of farmers on off-farm inputs."[15]

When first learning about the food system, I thought there must be a simple solution — just get all the farmers to stop using chemicals. They certainly would change if they understood the dangers and long-term effects. Well, that was about as naive as it gets. Many farmers I have met over the years want to be better land stewards than the most radical environmentalists, but most of them feel imprisoned by this downward spiral. The pressure to compete for less and less of the consumer's dollar and still pay off their debts is enormous.

> **"As a nation, we spend only about ten percent, or a dime out of each dollar, of our disposable income for farm produced food."**

On the consumer's side, we haven't seen much change in terms of the cost of food. Sometimes meat or fish seems to skyrocket, or new fancy foods seem out of our budget, but in general the staples have stayed at about the same prices.

Behind the scenes, however, prices are changing significantly for those who produce. According to agricultural economist and sustainable agriculture advocate, John Ikerd, "As a nation, we spend only about ten percent, or a dime out of each dollar, of our disposable income for farm produced food. Equally important, the farmer gets only a single penny out of that dime, while nine cents goes to the marketing and input firms. We now pay more for packaging and advertising than we pay the farmer to produce the food."[16]

Now this really bothers me. I can see how the excessive packaging for processed foods is a ridiculous waste. But what about the meat counters where there is no packaging, or egg cartons that haven't changed in many years? Somehow I don't think it really is all packaging and advertising. Somebody is making money, and it is not the farmer.

The fact is that a very few companies are making most of the money. Over the years, a handful of transnational corporations has bought up the little (and not so little) guys to control most of the category. Wisconsin law professor Peter Carstensen indicates that these companies have a pricing advantage over farmers and ranchers. He reports, "The spread between prices paid for livestock and the wholesale price of meat has widened in the past few years by 52 percent for pork and 24 percent for beef."[17] Well, that explains the meat counter.

The process of companies buying up categories, such as beef, is referred to as horizontal integration. Another system that has reared its ugly head is known as vertical integration: when one large company buys as many of the functions as possible for getting food from farm to fork. Most of these functions are found at the processing companies, such as slaughterhouses or storage units. "Like the narrow opening of an hourglass which controls the flow of sand from the top to the bottom, the processing firms are positioned between thousands of producers and millions of consumers in the United States and the world. These firms have a disproportionate amount of influence on the quality, quantity, type, location of production, and price of the product at the production stage and throughout the entire food system."[18]

Going hand in hand with vertical integration is contract farming, where growers really start to look like the serfs in this agricultural system. One large firm will contract with a farmer to grow grain or vegetables, or raise beef, pork, or poultry under certain specifications. But these specifications are very tight, many times calling for investments in certain equipment (which, of course, puts the farmer further in debt) or in seed that comes directly from the contracting company.

This type of farming, describes writer William Greider, "begins to resemble a fast-food franchise to run a burger joint or an auto dealership. The operator buys the supplies and equipment from the brand-name company and produces to its uniform specifications."[19] The only thing the company does not take care of for the grower is risk. Everything else seems regulated, down to when the product is shipped and where it is stored. In some cases, the company will send "specialists" to review the growing or raising practices to "assist" with any difficulties. Greider writes, "Richard Levins, an agricultural economist at the University of Minnesota, said these production contracts covered about $60 billion by 1997, almost one-third of farm-level crop and livestock sales, and expanded greatly since. Mainstream authorities regard supply contracting as the future."[20]

Thankfully, many people are working toward change. The US office of the Rural Advancement Foundation International (RAFI-USA) has a Contract Agriculture Reform Program underway. It is an effort to ensure that contract arrangements between individual farmers and processors are fair and equitable. Its primary focus is on the poultry industry, one of the worst in terms of contracts.

Contract agriculture is becoming further and further embedded in our system, in part due to an inequitable farm subsidy in the US. The consolidation of the farming industry feeds a serf system, as described in a recent *New York Times* article: "Because large farmers receive the largest subsidies, they are buying out smaller farmers, leading to what the Agriculture Department calls a 'rapid decline' of family farms under 100 acres and the rise of old-fashioned tenant farming. Over three-fourths of rice farms are worked by tenants or part-owners, the [Agriculture] department says."[21]

Rice farming has been under some surveillance since the Environmental Working Group set up its website listing all the farms receiving subsidies and exactly how much they get. (This move has caused a much-awaited increase in awareness! Check it out at **<www.ewg.org>**.) Three of the top five subsidy payments went to rice farms, all in the same region of Arkansas, for a grand total of $92.6 million over five years.[22] Ownership of at least one of the three sounds as if it was set up specifically to garner the greatest payment. As reported in the *Washington Post*, "Its 39 owners are organized into 66 separate 'corporations,' an arrangement that allows the farm to maximize benefits under allowable payment limits and also limits owner's liability...."[23]

Farm support programs have existed since the early 1930s, when approximately one-quarter of the population was still living on farms. The price supports and direct subsidies (cash payments to growers from our government) were intended to stabilize the agricultural sector while at the same time ensuring an abundant and inexpensive food supply.[24]

Today those numbers look very different. As we discussed earlier, only two percent of the US population lives on farms, and the gap between the rich and poor farmers grows ever wider. According to a USDA report from September 2001, current payments don't find their way into the pockets of the needier farms. "The most financially disadvantaged farm today is the low-income, low-wealth group. This limited-resource group comprised about 6 percent of farms, had average household income of $9,500, but received less than 1 percent of direct government payments in 1999. In contrast, 47 percent of payments went to large commercial farms, which contributed nearly half of program commodity production and had

> "Subsidies are usually tied to production, so larger farms with larger output get larger payments."

average household income of $135,000."[25] These farms make up less than 10 percent of the total. Sixty percent of American farms receive no crop subsidies.[26] Subsidies are usually tied to production, so larger farms with larger output get larger payments.

We were supposed to watch farm subsidies begin to phase out altogether. Farm legislation passed in 1996 was intended to lower subsidy levels. In the 1980s, subsidies averaged $15 billion yearly. By the 1990s, an improved market and economic conditions prevailed, and outlays dropped to approximately $10 million per year. By 1996, with new legislation, the projected payments were forecast to run at $6 million a year.[27] Through a variety of emergency funding laws, in response to decline in commodity prices and natural disasters, payments actually increased substantially. "For calendar 2000, direct farm payments reached a total of $24 billion — a figure representing over one-half of net farm income for the year."[28]

I would love to tell you a happy ending to this story, but at the moment the players are all gathered on Capitol Hill, working it out. The good news is that there will be change. How that change will turn out for the majority of farmers, it's too soon to tell. In the meantime, support those not getting those supports: buy from your local grower.

Shopping tip

"In the meantime, support those not getting those supports: buy from your local grower."

5

The Great and Powerful Consumer

FARMERS HAVE FACED INCREASING PRESSURES OVER THE YEARS. We expect them to be agronomist, entomologist, pathologist, soil scientist, marketer, business manager, environmentalist, etc. Now we say, "In the face of corporate pressure to do otherwise, please change everything you've learned about growing our food, and do it all without your tools." It is a bit like telling an artist to paint without a brush or a carpenter to build a house without his hammer and nails. It's not that it can't happen. It just might help to have patience and encouragement from us.

The power of upfront investments

I'm not advocating for a stock market approach, but the age-old theory of early investments applies to the local grocer, manufacturers, farmers, and a slew of other agriculture types. When we signal to the produce buyer by spending more for organic or IPM grown, we get the word to farmers that we think it's worth their efforts to grow with the Earth in mind. When we tell McDonalds we don't want GMOs in our fries, it can work, to a certain extent. McDonald's has asked its potato suppliers not to use genetically engineered spuds, but the potatoes are still fried in oil from gene-spliced soybeans.[1] Two steps forward, one step back.

Gerber Baby Food has said no to GMOs and yes to organics. "I have got to listen to my customers. So, if there is an issue, or even an inkling of an issue, I am going to make amends. We have to act preemptively," said Al Piergallini, president of Novartis's (Gerber's parent company) US consumer health operations.[2] Consumers do make a difference! Home Depot is selling sustainable forestry certified wood products, Starbucks is importing some organic, shade-grown coffee. More and more companies see the writing on the wall. Consumers want it! That is all well and good as long as we truly do want it. We do have the power to signal the system, but only if we put our money where our mouths are.

> ### Shopping tip
>
> *"When we signal to the produce buyer by spending more for organic or IPM grown, we get the word to farmers that we think it's worth their efforts to grow with the Earth in mind."*

My favorite comment from a powerful influencer on the food system came from former Secretary of Agriculture Dan Glickman when he answered reporters in 1999 on the fate of GMO labeling. He said, "Frankly, if the consumers demand labeling ... we're probably going to end up with a labeling scheme." It hasn't worked out that way ... yet. But we have not yet made as much of a demand as in Europe. The point is, we can demand a healthy food system for our bodies and our Earth. And as we do, I believe eco-foods will snowball.

> **"The point is, we can demand a healthy food system for our bodies and our Earth. And as we do, I believe eco-foods will snowball."**

At our public universities

Once the signal has been sent, all sorts of efforts may take off. One such effort will certainly be more research in the area of organic farming. At this point, the USDA spends significantly fewer dollars on organic research than on biotechnology research. When my tax dollars are diverted away from a method of farming I appreciate to one I do not, I find it extremely frustrating. As sales figures for natural products increase (as a result of our spending), there is greater interest in doing this research. We can affect so much with our buying! The USDA does support some alternative farming programs, but they are still few and far between. Last year, one government budget line allowed for proposals from the alternative community (USDA Initiative for Future Agriculture and Food Systems), and a number of exciting, creative and progressive proposals emerged.

Thankfully, some wonderful programs received some funding, but the pot was very limited. It was hard to watch so many worthwhile groups vying for so few dollars. In fact, only two non-governmental organizations received funding from that pot in the end.

Research at land grant universities, the 67 national educational institutions that have a mission and receive some public funding to "serve the public good," has been minimal in the area of organic agriculture practices. A report from the Organic Farming Research Foundation said, "Out of nearly 886,000 acres of research land in the land-grant system, only 151 acres was set aside for organic research."[3]

University professors in agriculture have, over the years, accepted small grants from corporations to test chemicals. Their unbiased opinions have been needed to help clear the way to national registration, since corporations need the results to prove safety and efficacy. Tenure (life-long jobs) at universities is often granted with an eye to how much funding the individual can bring into the university. So the pressure is on the professor to accept donations.

In some cases, a university will package and sell research to corporations. Some sell the right to learn results of certain research before their competitors; others simply conduct research to aid the approval process. Most of this type of work is propriety-based. Stories about intellectual property rights and conflict of interest have increased over the years.[4] So I ask myself, why is a public university, paid for, in part, by tax dollars, doing research that is ultimately "for the corporate good" versus the "public good"? Many would argue they are the same.

Organizations are leading efforts to influence the research agenda at land grant universities. The California Sustainable Agriculture Working Group embarked on an exciting campaign to increase state funding for on-farm organic and sustainable agriculture research and education projects through the California Biological Agriculture Initiative. In May of 2001, the California State Assembly added $5 million for sustainable agriculture research and extension to the University of California's 2001–2002 budget.

A newly formed group, the Northeast Organic Network, is made up of farmers, researchers, extension educators, and grassroots non-profits working together to improve organic farmers' access to research and technical support. Funded with a $1.2 million USDA grant, the project takes a truly comprehensive approach to research, developing baseline levels with farmers and integrating farm and field data. Some of the universities on the network include the University of Maine, Rutgers University, and Cornell University.

Many wonderful people at colleges and universities are doing fabulous work. A case in point is Ron Prokopy, entomologist extraordinaire. His passion for understanding the behavior of notorious apple pests in the Northeast is mind-boggling. Since the early 1970s, Ron has worked to provide alternatives to chemicals. He has written more academic journal articles on the ways of IPM than he has shelves to hold them all. And he has been an integral part of the University of Massachusetts IPM apple team, a multidisciplinary group of researchers working to reduce reliance on chemicals.

This year, in the midst of improved awareness of the need for alternatives to our growing methods, the IPM program in Massachusetts is facing another cut in funding from the state. Unfortunately, neither corporations nor consumers wildly demand IPM, so funding is virtually nonexistent. Our state tax dollars may be removed from this program that ultimately serves "the public good."

Like Ron, many people at universities across the country are struggling to fight for bigger budgets, working with Community Supported Agriculture farms to do some research on a shoestring or developing new farmer programs with immigrants. From the University of California at Davis on the West Coast to the University of Maine at Orono on the East, more and more sustainable agriculture or farming alternatives programs are emerging at universities. Anything we can do to provide encouragement, from influencing state or local funding to making those everyday eco-food choices, will ultimately send messages loud and clear.

"We will now have organic standards that mean something because of the individuals who took the five minutes necessary to say, no thanks, please try again."

On top of Capitol Hill

If we cannot turn over the family nest egg to signal farmers, we can use our voices ... from sending pre-prepared postcards to our favorite politicians to asking our local grocery store managers to carry certain products. The US system of government is a democracy, and we do have the opportunity to influence politicians. Letters and postcards can make a significant difference. When the national organic standards first came out, there were several problems with them. You would think once the USDA had spent all this time drafting the standards and trying to appease everyone, that the debate would hardly make it to a podium. But with over 275,000 letters and postcards to the USDA over a couple of months, the bureaucratic behemoth turned around and worked with the organic community to do it right — real revisions with significant input. We will now have organic standards that mean something because of the individuals who took the five minutes necessary to say, "no thanks, please try again." There are many examples of these success stories. The difficulty is believing we can make a difference and then stepping up to the plate.

Since the 1990 Farm Bill, the sustainable agriculture community formulated its own lobbying effort on Capitol Hill. It exists on a shoestring budget and is supported by voluntary efforts of the organizations it represents. In comparison, expenditures for lobbying and campaign financing from the multinational corporations (shown in the following chart from the book *Bitter Harvest*), many of which profit greatly from the current industrial agriculture model, are significant. The Chemical Manufacturers Association, for example, spent $5,020,000 on lobbying. Let's look at company spending by category[5]:

CATEGORY	LOBBYING	CAMPAIGN FINANCING	DEM.	REP.
Chemical manufacturing	$29,975,745	$3,787,272	22%	78%
Agricultural services	$10,852,887	$3,548,542	36%	64%
Food processing and sales	$ 9,401,655	$5,785,834	38%	62%
Crop production	$7,625,143	$5,233,232	41%	59%
Food and beverage	$5,830,620	$4,805,948	29%	71%
Dairy	$1,451,744	$1,263,146	38%	62%
Livestock	$1,182,000	$1,400,867	28%	72%
Fisheries and wildlife	$ 992,710	$ 94,070	39%	61%
Poultry and eggs	$ 490,000	$ 624, 139	29%	71%

The National Campaign for Sustainable Agriculture was formed right after the 1990 Farm Bill. Recognizing the problematic farm policies in the bill, member organizations of the Midwest Sustainable Agriculture Working Group (MSAWG) initiated a call to action across the country to create the National Coordinating Council for Sustainable Agriculture. Their first task was to develop a national dialogue, where diverse organizations' desires for policy change could be voiced and integrated into a set of priorities for the 1996 Farm Bill. Representatives of each regional SAWG and many national groups met in Washington to finalize the proposals and set priorities for a National Campaign for Sustainable Agriculture.[6] A great deal of organizing and mobilizing went into those first six years.

I can call

Okay, so I never actually made the calls until last week ... and just now, I finished a phone call with my husband, pleading, "Please call our senators, it's easier than you would think." Yes, it's true. I cannot count myself one of the hundreds of thousands who called about the organic standards. I was simply too afraid. "How can this be?" you ask. Well, because I had never attempted to do the committed citizen thing before, I just didn't know any better. I was concerned that whoever was at the other end of the line would ask me a question. I knew so little – how would I ever answer them? They would know I was ignorant about political lingo and would chuckle around the water cooler for days. (No paranoia there, of course.) To avoid admitting this to myself, I conveniently adopted the cynical belief that one couldn't affect the political system with a little old phone call.

What changed my life? At a recent conference, I shared my fear with Kathy Lawrence of the National Campaign for Sustainable Agriculture. She affirmed my anxiety and guaranteed that lobbying efforts would be painless. "Simply read from the e-mails we send you," she said. "They won't ask you questions, I promise." So I put myself in her hands and made the calls.

The first person I reached knew less about the issues than I did, which was virtually nothing. I was able to tell him that I simply wanted money to go to small farmers, not to huge agribusinesses; and that I wanted importance placed on the environment. Okay, now I was on a roll. The next call was simply a message. Drat, how I wish we had more than two senators – I kind of liked this thing, after all.

Yesterday we got an e-mail from the National Campaign, with the heading, *"Your calls resulted in TWO MAJOR WINS last week!"* (Now I am doin' the dance!) followed by, *"Your calls on the remaining amendments are essential!"* I felt like the cowardly lion in *The Wizard of Oz*, receiving the medal for courage. "Let me at 'em!" I said out loud. So today, it's back to the senators with new requests, and it's old hat. All my friends and loved ones have been cajoled into making calls, too.

We can make a difference, each and every one of us. Just make the call. Really, you don't have to be an expert – you'll see!!

A variety of environmental conservation programs and alternative agriculture market programs became a part of the 1996 Farm Bill, in no small part thanks to this dynamic effort. Today the National Campaign has become a fixture in the policy work of Capitol Hill. During the current round of Farm Bill negotiations, it sent dozens of "Campaign Alerts," urging individuals to call their local senators and congressmen, and to enlist friends and neighbors in the effort. Responding is not as difficult as you might think; the Campaign makes it easy to participate. Sign on at **<www.sustainableagriculture.net>**

WEBSITE

Another opportunity is to get on as many group mailing lists as possible. They will keep you up to date with the issues of interest. In many cases, they will send you the pre-prepared postcards and tell you specifically what might help the cause. Throughout this book, I introduce a number of organizations doing great work. (Chapter 20 lists many of them.) Choose a handful and get connected! You can make the difference.

If organizations and politicians just aren't your thing, try influencing your local grocer. One large supermarket chain in the Northeast found responding to special requests was the easy part; letting customers know about their good deeds was another thing. Mike Messer (introduced in Chapter 1) is the general manager of the Hadley, Massachusetts Stop and Shop, an Ahold company, one of the big five supermarket multinationals in the world. With centralized warehousing, ordering and the like, Mike doesn't have a huge influence on what the store sells. However, he can make requests, and he does. He knows his store is located in a five-college town, and the sales of organics and other natural foods are high in this community. That in itself is still not enough to increase the proportion of these products. What is enough, he says, is a series of requests from consumers. "If I get a number of requests for a specific item or type of item, such as antibiotic-free chicken, I will respond." Mike has worked hard over the past year or so to increase locally grown foods. He has invited local growers to put on demonstrations and sell foods in the store. He works with, Community Involved in Sustaining Agriculture (CISA), a local group (see Chapter 6) to identify local foods with special signs throughout the produce section. It is not happening all the time, and more could be done. But it certainly is a start.

> **"Tell your friends and neighbors when your local store honors your request for eco-foods. Make requests, then make a big deal when they are honored."**

So sometimes just telling your closest friends and neighbors — that word-of-mouth thing — can be the best support you can give. Tell your friends and neighbors when your local store honors your request for eco-foods. Make requests, then make a big deal when they are honored. We can change this system, one request at a time.

6

Don't Worry, Buy Local

If communities of farmers and consumers wish to promote a sustainable, safe, reasonably inexpensive supply of good food, then they must see that the best, the safest, and most dependable source of food for a city is not the global economy, with its extreme vulnerabilities and extravagant transportation costs, but its own surrounding countryside.

— WENDELL BERRY

THE CLOSER THE FOOD SOURCE, THE BETTER FOR THE EARTH, our neighbors, and our farmers. Buying food grown near home is one action we can take that makes sense for us and cents for our farmers. From field to fork, each step away from the source adds a bit more cost, more energy, and potentially more chemicals. Shorten the distance, lessen the cost and waste, support your neighbor, and save valuable open agricultural land.

Unfortunately, buying locally is not that easy, and it can result in an endorsement of the use of chemicals. If your local grower uses production methods you're not happy with, is it necessarily the best choice? Then there is the neighbor on the other side of the globe to think of — doesn't that farmer deserve as much access to a market as your neighbor down the road? And finally, there is the hard-to-avoid deterrent to local eco-eating: our universal desire for fresh fruits and vegetables out of season, just when they are more attractive from somewhere else.

How did we get here?

It is often said that our focus on the world economy has moved us to a principle of "distance and durability." This has become as true for food as for other products in the industrialized world economy. But how did this happen? How did we get so far away from our food sources? From plant to plate, our food travels an average of 1,300 miles and is passed through the hands of at least six different people, a lot of fingerprints on the average apple. How did we get into a food system where the orchard up the road supplies another state, and our pies are filled with tree fruit from the opposite coast?

Kate Clancy from the Henry A. Wallace Center for Agriculture and Environmental Policy at Winrock International frames the historic progression. "In the decades between 1820 and 1870 farmers in the Northeast saw the markets offered by large cities like New York and Boston and started to produce for those markets. This marked the shift from regionalism to nationalism, and was aided by technologies like the mower and reaper, the settling of the West, and the development of the railroad. By the end of the 1870s agriculture had replaced mining and ranching as the major economic force in the West, and agricultural specialization occurred throughout the country. As nationalism grew, middlemen increased to accommodate the food coming to the East by rail and steamer. Domination by wholesalers posed marketing problems for local farmers — it was about 1920 that the New York City market for Northwest apples was developed to replace New York state apples. Local growers were not producing the volumes needed to compete with farmers in other parts of the country, and by 1924 only 5 to 10 percent of the food supply of New England was locally produced."[1] This statistic seems entirely in contrast with the image of the pilgrims sitting around that first Thanksgiving table sharing the bountiful harvest of New England. On the other hand, today there are a lot more tables and many more mouths to feed.

We have come, in a fairly short period of time, from localism to regionalism to nationalism, and — now that our government has agreed to international trade relations through the North American Free Trade Agreement (NAFTA), and the General Agreement of Tariffs and Trade (GATT) — globalism. We eat food grown all

Shopping tip

"Buying food grown near home is one action we can take that makes sense for us and cents for our farmers. Shorten the distance, lessen the cost and waste, support your neighbor, and save valuable open agricultural land."

over the world. It sounds rather cosmopolitan on the surface, and not such a bad thing. The mystique of mangoes and daikon radishes is revealed on our grocery shelves on a continuous basis, invoking a scene of expanding the harvest table and sharing with our neighbors around the world. If equity were in play — where the equation for imports and exports were similar in all parts of the country or around the globe — it would be a wonderful scene.

When trade comes up in discussion, we usually worry about the small Southern Hemisphere countries. We think that without the miles of agriculturally productive land that we have in the United States, these small islands of crop specialization will certainly become stuck in the importer web, constantly sending out what little they can grow for a minimal cash return instead of focusing on feeding their own small populations through intensive subsistence farming. The conversation always seems to focus on the little guys (the underdogs), and yet some numbers show that maybe it is time we woke up and smelled the coffee, since our own dependency on imports has grown. A 1999 report to the National Farmers Union states, "About one-third of the vegetables consumed in this country are imported. The United States is also a net importer of beef."[2] So much for home on the range. What happened to our own cornucopia? It is not that we don't have the means to grow our own food. We are also a large exporter, but we have just chosen someone else's fare.

> "The United States is also a net importer of beef. It is not that we don't have the means to grow our own food. We are also a large exporter, but we have just chosen someone else's fare."

And who wouldn't? Some of the choices coming from other countries are very enticing: raspberries and cream at Christmas, clementine oranges in lunch boxes during mid-winter cold season, or crunchy sweet red peppers in salads in early spring. As Joan Gussow said, "Already during certain seasons, 70 percent of selected fruits and vegetables we choose from supermarket produce bins and restaurant menus are imported from developing countries."[3] Again, this might open the door to all sorts of new recipe ideas, if we all agreed to the same guiding and growing principles, such as environmental and child labor laws. Knowing that a five-year-old picked that cucumber instead of playing all day makes it much less refreshing to the palate.

Another concern about global food is the difference in health standards among producing countries worldwide. "Commenting on an outbreak of diarrheal disease caused by imported raspberries, a *New England Journal of Medicine* editorial pointed out that we are now eating raw fruits and veggies grown in places where US travelers are instructed to avoid foods that can't be peeled or cooked," Gussow continued.[4] Does this mean we should eliminate anything grown outside the US? Probably not. It means that awareness of where the food is coming from and the practices used in growing and processing it should be part of our buying decisions. Those tomatoes and peppers I almost bought in Chapter 1 were grown in Israel using I-don't-know-what-kind-of-growing practices.

> ## Shopping tip
>
> *"... awareness of where the food is coming from and the practices used in growing and processing it should be part of our buying decisions."*

One reason for the angry demonstration in Seattle against the World Trade Organization (WTO) and the international trade agreements was the potential for irresponsibility on the part of big business when the borders were opened. Some of this has clearly been realized. According to Gary Valen, "Since the signing of the NAFTA, more vegetable operations are moving to Mexico and other southern countries where agricultural chemicals are not as regulated as in the US."[5] See Chapter 8 for more on cross-border trade.

If we try to watch extra carefully the practices of those countries where our winter is their summer, will that be enough? Well, not really. Growing conditions in certain parts of the US can produce our summer fare out of season. For example, California now supplies more than 40 percent of US fresh produce.[6] Now there is the answer … for Californians. California is a state within our national borders with like-minded social agendas and responsible health practices. If you live in California, you have it made. If you live on the other side of the country, it is not so great, as it takes three times as much energy to truck a head of lettuce from California to New York as it does to grow it.[7]

Transportation costs in unexpected ways

From trucking to airplane delivery, non-renewable resources — specifically oil and gas — gobble up your hard-earned grocery bill. How much can it cost? In 1981, the Rodale Institute did a very thorough study of the US food system. At that time they estimated, based on US Department of Agriculture figures, "Americans paid almost $16 billion in 1980 to move their food around."[8] In the 20-plus years hence, that figure can only have grown. Some more fun facts on transport from that study: "The 4 million trucks (used primarily to transport food) travel annually 45 billion miles, a

Confessions of a Holland pepper purchaser

Now all of this "buy local" stuff is well and good. I truly want to be an eco-eater with sustainability in mind. Sometimes, however, it is just plain difficult. One of the demons I battle in the land of local is the Holland pepper, that perfectly ripe, brilliant red/orange/or yellow, always crunchy megasource for vitamin C. It is rare for me to get a good source of C. Neither my stomach nor my son's little tummy does well with acidic foods such as oranges and other citrus fruits. Watching him writhe in pain from gas bubbles tells me some sources of health are better than others for his little body. So when my children happily crunch away at their red peppers from Holland, I am truly in conflict mode.

These peppers are fresh as fresh can be, picked in the field and flown overnight. The Dutch go to great lengths to get their colorful gems into our produce sections within a blink of an eye. But then, there is the airplane fuel and what that costs our Earth ... and with each purchase, we send our dollars halfway around the world, taking a market away from local growers. Oh, bother! There is never a dull moment in this conscience of mine, always working at breakneck speed to figure out what is good for the Earth.

Today my son has a cold, the local season for red peppers has past, Holland peppers are on sale, and I happen to be going to the big supermarket. So don't be surprised to find a few peppers hiding underneath all the otherwise local eco-foods in my basket.

distance equal to 242 trips to the sun! Food trucks burn up $5.5 billion worth of fuel each year, expel over four million tons of pollutants into the air, and cause millions of dollars of damage to public highways."[9] These are truly jaw-dropping figures. If we stayed closer to home for supper, think how much we would save, in all sorts of ways.

Michael Shuman, a relocalization activist, identifies government transportation subsidies as the primary culprit in the enhanced transportation game. According to his research, "The national highway subsidy totals about $25 billion annually. Strip away subsidies to oil, roads and transport vehicles, impose green taxes on these activities to cover the environmental costs, and suddenly long-distance trade is no longer such a great bargain."[10] No one wants his or her own transportation to be curtailed. Thanksgiving wouldn't be the national travel holiday if it weren't for roads. And although we may be attracted to the Amish system of visiting only where you can go via horse and buggy, it seems our highway system is pretty entrenched.

On the other hand, any taxes or other discouragement to wasteful food transport we as citizens can encourage would be another endorsement for your farmer neighbor down the street. Such activity might also help to minimize the overuse of non-renewable, global-warming energy sources. It has been pretty well agreed at this point that our overuse of cars and trucks is a primary cause of our dramatic weather patterns. "The United Nations-sponsored Intergovernmental Panel on Climate Change, which represents 2,500 scientists from around the world, suggests that current trends of fossil fuel will release enough carbon dioxide into the atmosphere to raise global temperatures 1.5 to 6 degrees Fahrenheit over the next century."[11] With that said, let's go to other effects of long-distance transportation.

What happens to our food on the road? If food travels, on the average, 1,300 miles from field to fork, that means 20 hours minimum spent on-road travel. All but the most dedicated of corn connoisseurs would accept that much flavor loss from picking to eating. (The sugar in corn begins to turn into starch as soon as it is picked. Corn right out of the field yields the sweetest flavor.) However, other factors, such as packaging and sorting, may extend that travel time to a few days. The sweetness of the corn has definitely been transformed into heavy starch at that point. And there goes the flavor.

For our natural produce to take a road trip, what has to be added to or removed from it? Jack Kloppenburg and Steve Stevenson of the University of Wisconsin paint that picture vividly in their landmark paper, "Coming into the Foodshed." "If food products must travel 1,300 miles before they are consumed, they must be sufficiently durable to withstand shipping. But durability and shelf life are too often realized at the expense of palatability and nutritional content. The denatured, deflavored, industrial tomato is but the best known exemplar of a process that has affected many fruits and vegetables. Consumption even of such 'fresh' produce has declined in favor of processed foods that depend on artificial flavors, stabilizers, emulsifiers, sweeteners, and preservatives for their appeal."[12]

There is little doubt something has happened to the taste of our foods, particularly fresh vegetables. A carrot from a grocery rarely elicits the response one has to a carrot from the ground. They almost seem like different vegetables — the tasty variety and the not-tasty variety. And what happened to the tomato, that beautiful, round, red, ripe ball of flavor and nutrition? Tomatoes clearly show the difference between a locally grown in-season fruit (yes, it is a fruit, not a vegetable) and a "distant and durable" replica. "Cardboard" is the word generally heard to describe that tomato taste. So what happened?

Some scientists have been trying to devise ways to "improve" ripening of our tomatoes. One story of a resultant discovery goes like this: "Union Carbide ... markets a plant regulator called Ethrel. It is a versatile substance, used on tobacco, cherries, apples, and tomatoes, among other crops. The manufacturers recommend that Ethrel be applied when 5–30 percent of a tomato crop is pink or red and the rest 'mature green.' Two to three weeks later the entire crop can be harvested when it is uniformly ripe. What the drug does is cause 'an early release of ethylene — nature's ripening agent.' There is a problem, however, when this is applied to a crop of tomatoes destined for the retail market rather than processing. Because it speeds up ripening, the tomatoes keep speeding until they rot, which may be the day after you buy them."[13] There are several stories of potential "improvements." I think I will just wait until my tomatoes are in season ... locally.

> ### Shopping tip
> *"Tomatoes clearly show the difference between a locally grown in-season fruit and a distant and durable replica. Cardboard is the word generally heard to describe that tomato taste."*

Open space

Why is it a good thing to support small farmers who keep land open? Why not just let them move to the areas where farming can be managed through corporate agribusiness? Besides taking away the culture and knowledge of farming from your children, it would also remove all that land devoted to crops or grazing cows. No more stopping roadside with the kids to watch lambs boinging in the spring. What would happen to all the open space? If history repeats itself, suburban sprawl and development would pave our favorite fields. Julia Freedgood of the American Farmland Trust wrote, "Between 1982 and 1992, every state in the nation squandered prime and unique farmland to urban sprawl at an average rate of 50 acres every hour of every day. The process of farmland conversion tends to be incremental with one farm going out of production here and another there. As a result, the cumulative loss is often unappreciated until the last remaining farms become islands in a sea of new development."[14]

As a city-dweller, this may seem a remote issue until you're out for a drive or a special trip. Driving through Lancaster County, Pennsylvania, expecting acres upon acres of Amish farmland and instead seeing new neighborhood developments in every direction, can be a rude awakening to this issue of sprawl. When we don't experience the "country" every day, it may be hard to imagine the impact of development.

At the same time, those who live in the proximity of sprawl may be lulled by its takeover. A few houses here or there may seem like an economic boom until another traffic light is needed at the corner or your favorite walk no longer affords the same peace and quiet. In focus groups run by the American Farmland Trust to understand citizen response to suburban sprawl, quality of life issues took center stage. Although participants cited the aspects of sprawl we immediately think of — loss of scenic beauty, increased air and water pollution, and loss of wildlife habitat — " ... increased congestion, a more hectic pace of life, increased crime and a lost sense of community" were actually the central and predominate concerns.[15]

Once the land has been developed, there tends to be no going back. We may find, after the fact, that these quality-of-life issues were bigger than we had anticipated, and we want our neighboring fields back. We may have had another farmer waiting in the wings, but once those houses are up, the land has gone. One solution being tried in many communities is "land trusts." Money is raised for a specific piece of land and held in trust until another farmer or environmental program is willing to purchase it, most often at less than market value. This is not an income-producing deal, unless you see open space as a form of income much more valuable than cash. It holds the land out of arm's reach of developers and is a wonderful opportunity to invest in a sustainable food system. Elizabeth Henderson, Northeast organic farmer and advocate, said, "For new farmers, access to land is critical: more farmland off the real estate market and held by community land trusts will give more young people the opportunity to start farming on slim resources."[16] And a positive feedback loop emerges: new farmers, growing more sustainably on land, make it unavailable for new housing.

Take back the bank: Reclaiming the local economy

A similar success cycle is played out when dollars stay in a community. When buying local at a farm stand, farmers' market, or community-supported farm (see

Chapter 17), you direct cash back into your town. Not only does that dollar stay in the community, it is the seed to grow even more resources at your local level. This is the economic multiplier effect. Again, Michael Shuman describes it best: "The expenditure of a dollar in a community generates more than just one dollar's worth of activity. A worker who receives a paycheck of, say, $500, might spend half on food and half on rent. The store that sold the food might use its $250 in revenue to buy more produce from local farmers, and the landlord might spend her $250 on electricity bills from the local utility. Every expenditure cascades into a larger number of transactions that enrich the community."[17] According to Shuman, this all breeds good things: less vulnerability to outside events, more ecological consideration due to increased self-reliance, more diversification of jobs. Like so many things in life, it's a spiral up, a positive multiplier versus a downward slide. The good news is that "more than 40 communities in the United States — and some 2,000 worldwide — now issue their own local money to promote local buying and selling."[18] Keeping dollars within the community by using special currency redeemable only at local businesses discourages its disappearance to other parts of the country (or world.) Often in the world of agribusiness, however, dollars flow out, leaving the community debilitated. This is another indicator of our unhealthy food system. For the big farms of the central states, and those on both coasts where direct marketing is not a viable alternative, the dollar flows out with the gems of the land, and then those gems come back with an even bigger price tag. Every time a big potato farmer eats his own harvest in the form of french fries from McDonald's, he actually supports several other communities but his own. As organic rancher and farmer Fred Kirschenmann put it in a talk given to a Biodynamic conference, "We sell a lot of raw materials produced with cheap labor which flows out of the community and we never see the value of that production, and then we buy back a lot of expensive value-added products."[19]

And it's not just money that leaves. Sometimes giving away local natural resources is what hurts communities the most. An example of efforts to combat this is in the area of overharvesting of forests, which has generated a whole movement,

> ### Shopping tip
> *"When buying local at a farm stand, farmers' market, or community supported farm, you direct cash back into your town. Not only does that dollar stay in the community, it is the seed to grow even more resources at your local level."*

"community forestry," using models to try to integrate sustainability so communities keep "enough" of their precious resources. One classic example of a community that did give away its viability is the story of Nauru.

"In 1900 phosphate was discovered on Nauru (a small Pacific island), and today as a result of just over 90 years of phosphate mining, about 80 percent of the island is totally devastated. At the same time, the people of Nauru have had over the past several decades one of the highest per capita incomes in the world." As the story goes, Nauru was found to have the very hard-to-find natural phosphate for fertilizing soils. Since our agricultural system depends on large quantities of the big three fertilizers, Nauru's stash was like a gold mine, and it has been worked with that value in mind. For many years, the small island nation was under first Australian, then German rule. During this time, the Nauruans received less than one seven-hundredth of the phosphate's value. After decades of negotiations, Nauru received its independence in 1968. Its inhabitants continued to mine the phosphate, but received its full return. Almost 30 years later, the people received an out-of-court settlement of $120 million Australian for restitution and restoration. But it is considered too late. The phosphate has been exhausted, leaving the land inaccessible to humans and totally unusable for agricultural purposes. As the use of 80 percent of their land became diminished, Nauruans also became totally dependent on imports, including water. "Over the course of a century, first foreigners, and then, after Independence, Nauruans reduced the useful part of their homeland to a narrow strip of coastal land. Their once vibrant and unique culture has been transformed into one dependent upon a market economy."

"In a very real sense the decision to mine Nauru is the same as developing a small piece of land in upstate New York for a housing subdivision, or to log a portion of a rainforest in Indonesia, or to build a golf course in Hawaii. As resources are used we simply move to another place and exploit the resources there .... The more of a natural world we eliminate, however, the more dependent we are on the manufactured world we have created: money cannot be converted back into extinct species or their destroyed ecosystems."[20] Imagine not being able to let your child play on the playground where the ground may cave in. In a real sense, it is like the river that is too polluted to swim in, or the quarry where rocks are too loose to climb, it always seems that someone will fix it ... eventually. Apparently it is too late for Nauru.

Local and sprayed versus distant and not

So should we always buy local? This is the big question: is it better to buy local products even when they have been grown with pesticides and herbicides? Or should we buy the lettuce from 3,000 miles away because it is a vote for organic? Do you support the local farmstand when you can see that the farmer grows corn in the same fields year after year, obviously depleting the soil? These are tough questions. And the more local grower groups that enter the marketplace with eco-labeled items, the more confusing it becomes. Do you buy grape juice from organic vineyards, thus helping the salmon in Seattle (as the label suggests), or buy it from your neighbor who preserves the age-old squishing ritual, but still uses chemicals?

> "Do you support the local farmstand when you can see that the farmer grows corn in the same fields year after year, obviously depleting the soil? These are tough questions."

Is it crucial to keep local dollars in town even though you really want those clementines from Spain? Maybe supporting the farmer and community in Spain is a good thing, if they are using ecologically sound and socially responsible practices. Mark Ritchie, a thoughtful and insightful advocate who runs the International Agriculture and Trade Policy organization, said, "One way that globalization of organic could help over the long term is if it raises the income of local community at both ends."[21] There is no question that no matter where the product is produced, there is a local community in that area. A recent e-mail discussion began over this very question among the Integrated Food and Farming System listserv. Almost everyone agreed that buying local instead of product from Thailand was the only sensible decision. However, one of the few alternative views came from Tim Bowser, now at the Kellogg Foundation's Fires of Hope project, who said, "I cannot justify abandoning this Thai farmer as my global neighbor." That has stuck with me and forced me to think about both sides.

There are no perfect answers to these questions. Social and environmental considerations abound, and the only solution is to weigh them against your own individual values. If the environment is your first consideration, Warren Leon, executive director of the Northeast Sustainable Energy Association, suggests that transportation and other "buy local" arguments may be less important to global degradation, but more important to social health. "By far, most of the environmental damage caused by food consumption comes from growing the food .... Because the cultivation process (versus the processing, packaging, and shipping) is the most important consideration, it is probably better for the overall environment to purchase organic broccoli grown locally. Of course, finding broccoli grown locally using the same organic cultivation methods would be the best possible solution. Besides, there are often reasons for buying local foods that have nothing to do with the reduced energy use that comes from not having to ship it long distances. The strongest arguments for buying locally grown food probably have to do with saving local farmland from development and supporting the local economy."[22] So the answer to the big question seems to be individual choice. Now, how do we get the information to make a wise selection?

What's happening?

Today many organizations are supporting your decision-making process with information and options. They are making sure access to local products continues to expand, and they are working hard to develop new ways to inform you of the source of your long-distance food choices.

National

For years, a great deal of the agricultural support, both verbal and financial, coming from our federal government has been about agribusiness, biotechnology, rural development and land grant research. Recently a new, small addition to the USDA library has added to the language of small farms and sustainability. "A Time to Act" is a report from the 30-member USDA National Commission on Small Farms, which looked at the structure of agriculture and its effect on small farms in 1996. Today the USDA has initiated a campaign to address the issues brought forward in the report.

The report articulated the findings and recommendations of the commission and sheds a hopeful light on the need to "buy local." Consider this excerpt:

> Amidst the dominant talk of a global economy are voices articulating the hope of a
> local or regional food economy where small farmers play a central role. In a local or
> regional food economy, small farmers produce for community food and fiber needs
> and sell their products through alternative marketing channels. The strength of a
> local food economy is the relationships between farmers and community citizens.
> Through this relationship, small farmers provide fresh, in-season food appreciated
> and purchased by community citizens. The relationship creates an opportunity for
> mutual trust and support, contributing to the betterment of the community as a
> whole.[23]

This report contains a number of recommendations for improving local agricultural marketing, such as developing programs for regional identity of products produced locally by small family farmers, or "eco-labels" to describe stewardship practices used in the production of the product and benefits to the environment. The report also endorses the USDA's previous efforts and asks for expansion of the farmers' markets project; the Women, Infants and Children/Farmers Market Nutrition Program; and food-stamp programs at farmers' markets and CSA farms. The report asks for assistance in opening up other local markets to small farmers, such as local school lunch programs and federal agency cafeterias, including national parks. Any opportunity we have, as citizens, to urge the USDA to support these programs will further our chances for a truly sustainable local food system.

International

While some countries are just beginning to label products with place or country of origin, others have had such programs for years and are now moving on to more creative opportunities. Certainly the European Union appears to have some of the most innovative local buying activities. "In Europe, a new food labeling system allows customers to know how many 'food-miles' produce has traveled."[24] In

> "In some countries, electronic kiosks are being added to grocery stores, where you can press a button to find out how and where the product was grown."

Europe, you can find the actual facts. In some countries, electronic kiosks are being added to grocery stores, where you can press a button to find out how and where the product was grown. A variety of "locally grown" products is making its way to local markets. One example of locally labeled meat is from Germany, where a 340-member cooperative of pork farmers, Schwäbisch Hällisches Schwein, work on an average of 75 acres each under strict production guidelines. When the local breed of pigs was endangered, the community began the initiative to support the revitalization of the species and its products.

In France, the Appellation d'Origine Controlee (AOC) label has been on the books since May 1919. It guarantees that a product has been produced within a specified region, following established methods of production, which are much more detailed than simply reducing chemicals. These farmers must use the same standards, right down to the milking tins. The AOC label is most often seen on wines and cheeses, and on some meat products. This is a country where localism and regionalism provide a true national source of pride. The agriculture reflects it. One of the interesting opportunities to buy local in France is the farmer/producer-run grocery store. Sixty shops dot the French countryside that makes up the AVEC (Agriculteurs en Vente Collective Directe) system. One of these stores is "Uniferme," located in the Rhone-Alps region in St. Andeol-le-Chateau. At least a dozen farmers run the store cooperatively, with each providing a specific niche category, such as poultry, dairy, or fruits. They rotate coverage of the store, so there is always a farmer to talk to. The selections are unbelievably fresh and are all grown within a certain geographic proximity.

Initiatives in other countries include regional park and farm collaborations and extensive agricultural tourism programs. Staying on a farm while you tour Europe certainly brings you closer to the essence of the countryside.

State

Many states are establishing campaigns to identify their products. "Virginia Fresh" or "Picked in Tennessee" are two such communications campaigns complete with labeling, flyers, and billboards. "Maine Farms" is one of several state programs focused on developing local agriculture. However, unlike most states where activity is funded through the governmental department of food and agriculture, Maine Farms is under the auspices of Coastal Enterprises Inc., a non-profit community development corporation. The project's purpose is to develop strategies for supporting Maine's small farmers and food processors. Similar to other local agricultural support organizations, it looks to developing value-added "fresh-processed" operations for Maine farm products; it supports small, local markets that encourage the sale of locally grown and Maine-made food; and it develops food policy programs to look at barriers and opportunities for the local food system and train new and existing farmers in innovations. More and more of these programs are popping up with better "communications with consumers" strategies supplying us with the reminder and incentive to buy locally grown.

Regional

Another such organization communicating in a very professional way is the Community Involved in Sustaining Agriculture. Facing such statistics as, "since 1945, agricultural acreage in Massachusetts has decreased by more than 1.5 million acres — an area twice the size of Rhode Island,"[25] a consortium of local politicians, farmers, academics from the local land grant university, consumers, and grocery store managers came together to develop a plan to market local agriculture to the citizens of Western Massachusetts. These efforts were funded as part of the W. K. Kellogg Foundation Fires of Hope project.

The campaign highlights the farmer's face and the role consumers can play in supporting local economies and maintaining the rural landscapes of the region. It has a multi-media advertising strategy that includes radio, newspaper, and bus sign advertising, direct mail, in-store tastings, appearances at fairs and festivals, point-of-purchase materials in area stores, a web page, and public relations.

In 1999, the first Local Hero campaign evaluation indicated success in increasing the purchase of locally grown food. A post-campaign phone survey conducted by Penn, Schoen and Berland Associates of Washington, DC found that 53 percent of those surveyed were aware of the campaign, and of those, 61 percent were influenced to buy locally grown food. Today, campaign materials are being distributed as a "toolkit" throughout the movement as a model for local endeavors, available at **<www.foodroutes.org>**.

WEBSITE

County

Going to the next smaller unit of activity is a campaign on the county level on the other side of the country in Auburn, California (north of Sacramento). PlacerGROWN is a marketing program to assist local agricultural producers. Its goal is to bring communities and people together for the support and growth of agriculture in Placer County. Like many of the other programs, it develops new markets with grocers, institutions, restaurants, shops and other stores. It also explores new tourism markets, promotes Placer County agriculture at fairs and community events, provides educational packets for the media, consumers, schools and the general public, provides stickers and point-of-purchase cards to identify PlacerGROWN producers, and promotes a harvest calendar which highlights a "Reason for the Seasons."

> "PlacerGROWN is a marketing program to assist local agricultural producers. Its goal is to bring communities and people together for the support and growth of agriculture in Placer County."

Thanks to these groups at all levels, more of us are becoming aware of locally grown or raised items. Now all we have to do is choose them.

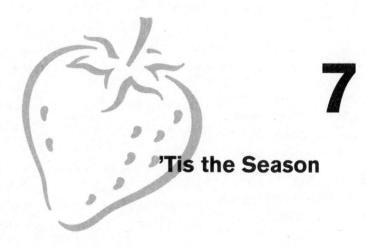

7

'Tis the Season

THOSE PILGRIMS HAD SOMETHING, CELEBRATING WITH SQUASH AND CRANBERRIES in November. Eating what's "now" means more than being fashionable; it's a healthy habit for all.

Eat what's ripe

It makes sense: whatever is coming out of the ground at the moment (if it is handled properly) is probably the best for us. No storing, preserving, or transporting to steal those precious nutrients. We intuitively know this when we look for freshness. Statistically, freshness is our top concern when buying produce. As writer Terra Brockman puts it, "Freshness is not just a fuzzy feel-good word of ad-speak. It is crucial. Studies show a steep decline in nutritional value from the moment produce is plucked from the field. If you eat it within 24 hours, you get significantly more vitamins and phytochemicals."[1] Most of us probably don't think of phytochemicals first.

Although the nutritional value of our food is important (and we will get to that later), we tend to associate freshness with flavor. Sometimes it is appearance that signals a far-too-long shelf life, but ultimately we are looking to satisfy the palate. I agree with author Fran McManus from Eating Fresh Publications, who says,

"Seasonal products taste better because they are fresher. When the weather turns brisk, the stomach cries for dishes that will warm the body and the soul. There are hearty vegetables that actually grow better and taste better in the winter months."[2] Give me a carrot well past the first frost any day. All that sugar seems to dart under cover and into the roots to escape the chilly air.

Although flavor remains the primary motivator in our food purchases, solving some of those food-system issues addressed in earlier chapters contributes to palatability. A local and seasonal food purchase is a vote for a positive solution and a step away from the industrial model of agriculture. Remember that most of that industrial model is devoted to extensive inputs, heavy processing, and too much energy. Laura B. DeLind states, "Not only does the system use 10–15 calories of energy to deliver one calorie of food, but processing, packaging, transportation, and marketing account for 75–85 percent of the energy consumed."[3] Buying local, seasonal whole foods removes many of these costs.

> "A local and seasonal food purchase is a vote for a positive solution and a step away from the industrial model of agriculture."

A study from the Leopold Center for Sustainable Agriculture in Iowa, "Food, fuel and freeways," examines closely some of these costs to the earth. The researchers used a "Weighted Average Source Distance" calculation to determine the average distance most foods traveled to Chicago (1,518 miles, up from 1,245 in 1981) and the average distance for local/regional food delivery to institutional destinations (44.6 miles.) From these figures they identified the amount of fuel and CO_2 emissions for comparison. Their results indicated that, "growing and transporting 10 percent more of the produce for Iowa consumption in an Iowa-based regional or local food system would result in an annual savings ranging from 294 to 348 thousand gallons of fuel, depending on the system and truck type … and would result in an annual reduction in CO_2 emissions ranging from 7.0 to 7.9 million pounds, depending on the system and truck type."[4]

> "Eating seasonally may be better for our souls."

All right, this is ridiculous. We are using all of this energy and emitting all this ozone-depleting gas just to get a head of iceberg and some flavorless red baseballs we call tomatoes in the dead of winter? This comment from Dr Joan Gussow of Columbia University sums it up nicely: "It is energetically insane to chill perishable produce and transport it thousands of miles across oceans and national borders so that we can have fresh yellow peppers in Boston — in February."[5]

Fluttermutter flutters in early summer

The children experience a cornucopia of flavors in early summer, from fresh strawberries – picked and eaten fresh, in shortcake, in homemade ice cream (thanks to farmer Karen), and of course in jammin' sessions – to a confusing choice of peas: eat the whole pod fat with peas, don't eat the fat pod, but do eat the peas inside, eat the thin pod with no peas, and finally, fluffernutter, the children's favorite decadent mixture of marshmallow and peanut butter, so cherished that they think even rye bread carries it well.

Stop the presses! How can a dedicated eco-eater allow fluffernutter when Mother Earth is providing so many great gifts? Well, sometimes I just have to let loose. Summer is a great time to celebrate – the warmth, the bounty of food, the slow migration out of homes and into each others' lives – and a time to simply play. What better way to play than with a fluffernutter sandwich at summer camp? If truth be told, I even splurged once on a loaf of white bread, a veritable sin in our house. However, once the loaf was gone, that was it. One can only get off the track for so long. So what to do with the remaining fluff? Try rye. According to my eight-year-old, if you can forget the caraway flavor, it's not so bad.

Okay, better for our bodies and better for the earth ... is there anything else? Yes! Eating seasonally may be better for our souls. "We are part of nature, and nature is part of us. Cooking with the seasons sustains a connection as old as our species .... When you eat local seasonal produce, you are ingesting something that basked in the same sun as you did, was bathed in the same rains, and thrived on the same air. Cooking with the season imparts fundamental blessings — flavor, nutrition, and a physical and spiritual connection to our farmers, our communities, our ancestors, and our earth."[6]

Since we will return to the scientific again in a few paragraphs, let's take a moment and reflect on this spiritual piece. Clearly, choosing our food comes from all sorts of impulses: a desire for superior taste, a concern for nutritional health, a need to nurture our families. For the most part, many of these impulses remain hidden under the more immediate day-to-day needs: get something fast that is quick and easy to make. Let's go, go, go. What can I throw in my child's lunchbox that is ready to go and still healthy? I say "for the most part," because this Wednesday before Thanksgiving I saw other impulses rise to the occasion. People seemed as harried as ever, and yet these deeper needs for carefully planned quality foods were expressed more vividly. "What do you mean there are no local brussels sprouts?" Even our very-large-grocery chain-store manager told me he had ordered his family turkey from a local farmer. "A free-range, antibiotic-free, and organic bird … I can't wait to taste it," he said. It reminded me that we truly crave these qualities, these choices, this lifestyle, and this relationship with our earth. We just don't seem to make the time, day to day. Like any solid relationship, this one takes time.

And like any relationship, it ebbs and flows. At times it seems to flourish and then to wither, only to be reinvigorated again under some unanticipated pressure. Clearly, we experience connections to our seasons. Experiencing this type of communion with our foodstuffs seems somehow right. On a more practical level, it is just plain fun. Eating seasonally gives us "the delightful anticipation of the season's first tomatoes or asparagus, and the wistful good-bye to the last of these treats every year," as put by writer Deborah Byrd.[7] I am not a lettuce lover, but in early spring when I can almost smell the growth of those tiny leaves, I say, "Bring on the rabbit food, as much as possible, please!" And late in November, when the community farm shares its last official bounty until next June, "wistful" doesn't come close to describing the sense of loss. So like any good roller-coaster relationship, eating seasonally has its ups and downs. But of course, it is better to have loved and lost than to never have loved at all!

For those of you who have had enough sentiment, we will get back to the scientific. Once again, we will meet some great heroes saving our food for us all.

And the experts say …

Nutrition researchers say a majority of us think of a healthy salad as iceberg lettuce and tomatoes, a tough commodity for Northern growers in November. But these same nutritionists are on the bandwagon to expand our repertoire and show us how eating seasonally is better for our health, our farmers, and our Earth. Over a decade ago, Dr. Joan Dye Gussow, Mary Swartz Rose, Professor emeritus and former chair of the Nutrition Education program at Teacher's College, Columbia University, and Kate Clancy, former professor of nutrition at Syracuse University and now director of the Wallace Center, wrote an article in the *Journal of Nutrition*

Education, first introducing the subject of eating for the earth versus eating only for our own health. Since that time, they have continued to endorse the message, and another colleague, Jennifer Wilkins, a nutritionist at Cornell University, has expanded on the message. I am sure many others have contributed to this movement of eating seasonal, local foods, but I have found their work to be most influential. Kate Clancy is now the director of the Henry A. Wallace Center for Agricultural and Environmental Policy at Winrock International. Her message has expanded to include many of the critical issues of a sustainable food system, especially in the area of policy development and reform.

Joan Gussow continues to devote herself to promoting seasonal and local eating. In the mid 1990s, Gussow and Wilkins began working together on the practical application of eating seasonally. Wilkins and her colleagues had explored consumers' attitudes towards local eating. She found consumers were "largely unfamiliar with several very common northeastern winter vegetables and showed poor understanding of what fruits and vegetables one should expect to find from local sources and when during the year." In the same study, 72 percent of respondents believed it would be necessary to import fruits and vegetables to get enough variety for a healthy diet in the winter.[8] Wilkins' study wasn't the only evidence of concern over nutritional adequacy. Gussow remembers giving a talk at Berkeley in the early days (1980) "where a well-known nutrition professor challengingly asked me where on earth I thought Iowans would get their vitamin C in winter. I would like to think I reminded him that settlers survived in Iowa long before the Florida Citrus Commission was founded and that Iowans probably got their vitamin C from apples, cabbage, and potatoes. But I probably didn't have the wit to give such an answer, because I was aware of how bizarre my suggestion seemed — even to me."[9]

So scientific analysis was necessary. Wilkins led the development of a Northeast Regional Food Guide, one that would cover all the basics of the USDA food guide pyramid, but would expand the selections to enhance the local food and agriculture system.

At the International Conference on Agricultural Production and Nutrition in 1997, Wilkins introduced the findings from a study examining the nutritional adequacy of the northeast regional diet. From an analysis of typical menus, Wilkins and Gussow found that, "with the exception of iron in the winter non-vegetarian diet, all diets provided at least 100 percent of the RDA for the macronutrients and for all the major or 'leader' vitamins and minerals …. Indeed, the levels of vitamin

Celebrating from leftovers

This Christmas we enjoyed one of the best feasts ever. Was it the additional gratitude for being with family a few months after September 11? It probably was, to some degree. Was it the added attention I gave to food because I was writing this book? Sure, that helped. Was it the inspiration of so many around me sharing stories of admiration for food well loved and presented? That definitely had an impact. And yet I am still convinced it was primarily because we ate food that had been stored away for winter.

Sitting down to plan a meal for ten, I tend to start with cookbooks. This year I started with a visit to the farm cooler and greenhouse, both filled with leftovers from the growing season. There were pumpkins and squash (too many varieties to name), cabbage (both red and green), rutabagas, carrots, beets, parsnips, celeriac, and daikon radishes. There was a little sorrel, kale, and parsley left in the field.

Granted, this was a not-yet-white Christmas, and it had been relatively mild. I don't think we would normally have had this much left, but every year seems to be "non-normal."

That's when I pulled out the cookbooks. It was a very different experience, starting with specific foods instead of the traditional. (Don't worry, I still had to make my mom's black lace cookies, or clearly it would not have been Christmas.) There is something truly wonderful about working with fresh foods, especially at a time of year when most people run to the grocers. I felt I had real riches to share.

On the day of the holiday feast, when my husband wanted an excuse to take a long-overdue walk with his niece, I sent them to the farm to cut the

C and E, beta-carotene (and by implication the other carotenoids) are present in levels well above those recommended .... In conclusion, consumers, and nutrition educators who teach them, should be confident that diets based on seasonally available foods in the Northeast can be both enjoyable and nutritionally complete."[10]

So there you go. I particularly appreciate academic research that goes to the heart of the matter and answers the question definitively.

kale. From the field to the fork, within minutes — literally! Almost everything came from the farm, except the chicken breasts. Lo and behold, our local supermarket had all-natural, organic chicken, with no antibiotics and labeled "Free Farmed" by the American Humane Association Thank you, Michael!

So, here's the multi-course menu:

First course:	Parsnip soup and fresh baguettes from our local bakery
Salad course:	Tomatoes (local hothouse), mozzarella, and basil (from my window plant)
Main course:	Stuffed chicken breasts with raspberry sauce (frozen from the farm)
	Warm red cabbage salad
	Sorrell, potato and onion tart
	Kale
	Wild rice
	Pickled beets
	Sweet potato pie
Cheese course:	Variety of cheeses and baguettes
Dessert:	Cranberry crunch (Massachusetts cranberries) with whipped cream

How did it turn out? To be totally honest, I had a slew of hors d'oeuvres beforehand, so no one made it to the cheese board. Also, I forgot to put out a couple of items, including the pickled beets. I'll probably never open a restaurant, but I do love to cook … fresh, local, and organic leftovers!

To live the dream

Now that seasonal eating was clearly shown to be more than sufficient from a nutritional aspect, Gussow needed to take the next step and examine the practicality of constructing and maintaining such a dietary lifestyle. To this end, she has invested her heart and soul in an attempt to prove it is possible to eat locally and seasonally. Both the chaos and gems from this experience are captured in her newest book, *This Organic Life: Confessions of a Suburban Homesteader*. Through her quest to truly live this diet, she found challenges one might expect, and others one might not anticipate. She talks about the issue of menu diversity in an interview in *Health* magazine in 1997: "'My God, we've had tomato sauce for 12 nights,' she tells the reporter. 'What can you do to make it interesting?'" Even as a non-homesteader, I find sticking with what's ripe sometimes challenging. Gussow's culinary skills, however, leave me in the dust. "They've had pasta with raw tomatoes, basil, garlic, and olive oil; tomato-water soup with tiny new potatoes and coriander; tomato sandwiches on crusty country bread; and chunky tomato salsa with black beans and fresh tortillas."[11] Her ability to extend a simple fruit through the demands of a 21st century palate seems substantially honed to me.

Gussow shares a couple of barriers to good eating in a 1999 report from the Iowa State University Extension. In it she states, "We are faced with an epidemic of culinary ineptitude and a universal sense of being time starved."[12] In my life, this is where the rubber meets the road. How, in our overextended lives, do we set aside time to make meals from scratch? I do not watch TV. And if I do, it is when I am in bed at 8:30 or 9:00 p.m. — one dopey sitcom and it's lights out for me. So how? I have worked through this issue by changing work schedules to accommodate my arrival at home to match the school bus, allowing for an extra hour plus to prepare meals and interact with my children. And it has become a blessing — a ritual of cozy-making, as my daughter calls it — of filling the house with the smells of fresh local harvests.

> "Eating seasonally requires stretching one's gastronomical muscles and getting in a rhythm of eating that is radically different from the way most of us procure, prepare and consume food."

As one member of Harmony Valley Farm, Wisconsin, put it, "Eating seasonally requires stretching one's gastronomical muscles and getting in a rhythm of eating that is radically different from the way most of us procure, prepare and consume food."[13] For me, this type of eating would not have come naturally. As my husband likes to remind me, I favored fettuccini alfredo and white bread (forget vegetables, fresh or otherwise) when we first met. I grew up with a seasonal shopper and experimental chefs as parents, so I had some awareness, but I had little interest in stretching. My culinary expertise improved over the years, but it was the farm, our Community Supported Agriculture (CSA) farm, that pulled me over the fence into the garden of delights. Forced to face kale and rutabagas and other strange new foodstuffs, I rushed to a myriad of cookbooks and farm-provided recipes. But since my most comfortable cooking comes from trying to replicate something I have had in a restaurant, it has been the chefs to whom I must tip my hat. And of course, many of these heroes hail from kitchens all over the world.

Thank goodness for the chefs

Enter hero number one: Alice Waters. She is one dynamite chef. Although I have never had the privilege of tasting her culinary creations, this woman has been a major inspiration out of the kitchen, into the fields, and back to the kitchen again. Her message has led the way for many chefs and individuals to cook with sustainable food. Referred to as "the doyenne of the create-your-menu-straight-from-the-garden movement, she says simply, 'They get it once they eat.' What they get is the intense flavor that comes from ingredients picked fresh and grown in a caring and respectful manner."[14] Alice Waters will admonish chefs and restaurateurs to "resist the temptation to serve any vegetable out of season."[15]

She has made an impact. Chefs from across the globe have redefined their creations by using what is available, now. A. J. Szenda, chef at the Plumed Horse in Saratoga, California, says, "I write my monthly menus around the fresh organic produce at the [farmers'] markets." For rising culinary star Charlie Deal, chef of Santa Cruz's year-old Oswald bistro, "Eating seasonally has just been instilled as the way things should be." He is proud of his track record. "We haven't bought any out-of-season products since we opened a year ago."[16]

Richard Ruben, New York chef and author of *The Farmer's Market Cookbook: Seasonal dishes Made from Nature's Freshest Ingredients* says, "there's nothing more exciting and flavorful than asparagus cut just an hour ago, as opposed to dried-out asparagus flown in from Mexico two weeks ago, it's like eating spring itself." Describing his approach as "in the moment, in the market" Mr. Ruben explains, "Today I went to buy fava beans, but I ended up with artichokes. They were at peak-season freshness, and therefore, much more enticing."[17]

Alexander Valley Vineyards Chef Jeff Young says, "I go out to the garden, and I'm like a kid in a candy store. It just doesn't get any better, when you go out and pick something and you're presenting it an hour later, and people say, 'How do you get the carrots to taste like this?' They're sweeter, tender, and more defined."[18] Not only do I feel desperate to jump into a car and drive the

> ## Shopping tip
> *"... there's nothing more exciting and flavorful than asparagus cut just an hour ago, as opposed to dried-out asparagus flown in from Mexico two weeks ago, it's like eating spring itself."*

3,000 miles to California for his carrot dish, I also feel grateful that so many wonderful chefs are modeling the behavior. These stewards of our palates have made a decision to enrich our lives through local, seasonal, flavorful food. It can't be easy to plan menus for the multitudes and find that Mother Nature has something else in store for you, literally.

And now the modeling has moved out of the confines of the white-tableclothed atmosphere and into our homes. "Season by Season" is a 22-part seasonal cooking program produced by public television station KQED and hosted by Chef Michael Chiarello of the celebrated Tra Vigne restaurant in California's Napa Valley. Each episode focuses on a particular foodstuff "in season," such as tomatoes or artichokes. The series' press release states, "More than a cooking show, 'Season by Season' uses food as a springboard for introducing viewers to a lifestyle that is in sync with nature, uncomplicated, and close to the ground… Visits with regional farmers and local makers of high-quality ingredients — an olive oil maker, an Arborio rice farmer — demonstrate the importance Chiarello attaches to knowing the source of your food." All right, it might be a press release, but I am still ready to do the dance. Hooray for the heroes — bring it on! (Read more about chefs in Chapter 18)

Finally, you might want to check out a few websites for seasonal eating tips. First, the Dane County, Wisconsin Farmers' Market at **<www.wisc.edu/agjourn/ dcfm/farmmarket/season.htm>** provides seasonal recipes and tips. Nutritiously Gourmet provides a list of foods in season on their site: **<www.nutritiouslygourmet.com/html/produce.html>**. American Farmland Trust has a nice chart at **<http://www.farmland.org/market/season.htm>**. Remember, of course, these are a sample of seasonal foods for those specific areas. You may have to do some digging to find what is right for your hometown. Have fun with the seasons!

8

You Can't Grow Coffee in Maine

NOT ALL PRODUCTS CAN BE GROWN AT HOME. So how do we choose from around the globe? Sometimes we might unknowingly get our pickings from elsewhere, as in the example of apples. Who would think, if you live an area where apples are grown, such as New England, that those "Delicious" red orbs at the local grocer flew 3,000 miles to get there? On the other hand, sometimes we clearly want something just not available at home. When oceans keep us from our neighbors, fair trade and equitable ethical practices become issues. Most of us just don't know how our purchases affect our neighbors around the globe or in our own country, for that matter. Thankfully, there are organizations working with some of the far-away sustainable farmers. From Fair Trade coffee growers to Rainforest Alliance bananas, lots of far-off friends are trying to ensure good quality growing practices for the food on our plates and the drink in our cups. What can we do to support them?

Apples crisscrossing borders

American apples grow from sea to shining sea, with 3,000 miles between each shore. To eat locally, we could stick to our own, but it seems we all have different tastes. Now add New Zealand, with its virtually pesticide-free fruit coming ripe at a time when our apples are rather mealy, and it is really tough to buy from home. Sometimes eating sustainably grown apples means choosing the best from the options offered. For a New Englander or eastern Canadian, that might mean apples grown within five miles in the fall, within the US or Canada for a couple of months, back home when the storage bins first open in January, back to the US for a few more months, and then maybe organic options from overseas. Is it worthwhile to eat on a schedule just to keep the earth in mind? You bet! Our buying sets the tone.

As with many other crops, the price of apples continues to decline while production costs escalate. As reported in the *New York Times*, "Red Delicious growers, for example, are receiving about 30¢ a pound for apples that cost up to 40¢ a pound to produce, though they sell for roughly $1 a pound in stores."[1] Apples spend a lot of time crossing international borders instead of simply staying at home. Recent US imports of apples were 301.5 million pounds, 94 percent of which came from Canada, New Zealand and Chile. US exports during the same time period were 1.6 billion pounds.[2] Growers complain of increased foreign competition, particularly from China, driving prices down. Although China is not one of the top three importers, its influence on the international market, particularly on processed apple juice, has had a major impact on North American growers. "By 1997, China produced more than four times as many apples as the United States. [As a result,] exports of Washington apples to Indonesia have declined about 80 percent in recent years."[3]

Washington state produces over half the nation's apples, nearly 60 percent. If you live in the Northwest region, you're in luck — you can eat apples locally from the number one producer state and feel good about it. (Of course, check the production practices. Apples often come with a great deal of pesticide residue.) If, however, you hail from the east, you may be spending a good portion of your apple-a-day dollar on transportation across 3,000 miles. New York state is the second largest apple-producing state. Participants at a 1997 international conference on agriculture were told, "According to a recent report less than 4 percent of all the apples produced in New York State go to the New York City fresh and processed apple market, which is now primarily served by other states and countries."[4]

The story of the New York state apple industry is a great example of how little we eat of our own. Thanks to a study put together by Laura Howard in 1995 for Mothers & Others for a Livable Planet titled, "Nibbling on Big Apple Market: Will Northeast Growers Retain or Lose Their Share of Local Markets?" we have a clear picture of what we are doing, or not doing, for our own region. "New York state produces about 28 million bushels of apples per year, making it the second only to Washington in state apple production in the United States. Yet despite the fact that the state's orchardists produce nine times the average quantity of apples utilized by the New York City market, three-quarters of the city's fresh apples come from Washington state, California, and overseas."[5] So now we understand, if we live in the East, there may be plenty to eat from the East; in the West, plenty from the West. What about the middle? If they don't produce as much as the coasts, they must already eat all they have. An interesting study looking at apple consumption in Iowa sheds further light on this perplexing problem.

The study in Iowa gave results similar to those of the New York analysis, just in smaller quantities. "Looking at fresh apple per capita consumption, Iowans eat almost 1.3 million bushels of fresh apples per year, but Iowa grows only about 15 percent of the fresh apples it consumes." The study dug a bit deeper by visiting grocers in season. "Produce department shelf space for apples was surveyed at eight supermarkets representing four different grocery chains in six Iowa cities (Ames, Ankeny, Cedar Rapids, Davenport, Des Moines, and Iowa City) from September 20 through October 3, 1999. The survey found that apples from Arizona, Illinois, Iowa, Michigan, Minnesota, Missouri, New Zealand, South Africa, Utah, and Washington were for sale. Iowa apples averaged less than 10 percent of the total apple shelf space across these stores." And it is not just the grocery stores with their centralized warehouse systems causing the problem. For example, "Iowa State University residence halls purchased 732 bushels of apples grown in other states from September to December, 1998."[6]

How does New Zealand keep coming up as a big apple exporter? They don't produce a particularly large quantity of apples, as China does. They do, however, bring North Americans fresh apples at a time when we are eating ours from the refrigerator. Most of the apples we see from Washington state have been harvested for controlled atmosphere storage, then distributed over time to extend the marketing season. As reported in *Good Fruit Grower* magazine, "Most apples in New Zealand are harvested, packed and cooled within 48 hours ... and sold in less than three months."[7] So they are fresh. They also come at the opposite of our harvest time — mid-February to mid-March — a time when many North Americans are bursting to get out and eat something from Mother Earth. They also bring us varieties we particularly like: Braeburns, Galas, and Royal Galas.

These apples have become, for me, a worthy exception to the principle of buying local. Not only do I love the taste of a good, fresh apple at a time when I loathe the winter, I also approve of their production practices.

The New Zealand Apple and Pear Board (ENZA) is the marketing arm that also regulates production practices and quality grades (such as percentage of red color). Currently the board requires all apple growers in the country to follow its Integrated Fruit Production Programme, or IFP, similar to a North American Integrated Pest Management program, IPM. Currently 10 percent of ENZA's growers are organic (Bio-Gro certified), and another 20 percent have begun the three-year process of conversion.

Now don't get me wrong, I do not advocate eating a New Zealand apple over a locally grown apple in season. I do, however, promote the idea of dedication to quality growing practices with reduced chemical inputs. Any friend of IPM or organic is a friend of mine. So you will have to make this call yourself. Do the production practices outweigh the local aspect? This is a very confusing question, one I had to battle with myself while working with Wisconsin potato growers. Do I support a potato grown under strict biointensive IPM standards from 300 miles away over a chemically produced spud grown next door? In their case, I went for production practices. Others may give priority to supporting local growers.

Shopping tip

"Now don't get me wrong, I do not advocate eating a New Zealand apple over a locally grown apple in season. I do, however, promote the idea of dedication to quality growing practices with reduced chemical inputs. Any friend of IPM or organic is a friend of mine."

Back to apples: as you may have guessed, there are heroes. For example, Dave Breen, the owner of Breen's IGA grocery stores in three upstate New York towns, posted a sign in his Williamson store saying, "No Washington-grown apples will be sold during the local harvest season."[8] You would think this would be a fairly easy store policy to live by, but when a customer wants an apple that is not quite ready in New York and the store next door has one from Washington, that owner could lose customers to the competition. It is a brave soul who stands up for the locally produced!

In the mid 90s, Mothers & Others launched a "CORE Values Northeast" program, labeling apples grown in the Northeast under approved growing practices, to highlight certain growers' dedication. At one of the kick-off events, Vermont's Deputy Commissioner of Agriculture, Roger Clapp, said, "The livelihoods of more than 100 Vermont apple farmers in the state who keep 4,000 acres in 'working landscape' are hanging in the balance, unless Vermonters stop buying inexpensive southern-hemisphere apples and the highly advertised Washington apples."[9] Yes, it is up to us!

What about those commodities that simply will not grow in our areas, the ones we couldn't buy locally if we wanted to? Coffee, chocolate, bananas, and citrus fruits are some of the top contenders. Let's start by looking at our favorite drink .

Equal Exchange and other coffee co-ops

We love our java. Coffee is so popular that it is the second most widely traded commodity in the world after oil, with the US being the largest consumer, importing more than 26 percent of the world's coffee or 2.45 billion pounds. Canada imports nearly 400 million pounds; 80 percent of US adults are regular or occasional coffee drinkers.[10] We can't grow it in our temperate climate, so how do we judge the validity of ecological choices from so far away? Over the past ten years, a variety of equitable justice and environmental organizations have led the way to ensure that Third World farmers using quality production practices receive their just rewards. Thankfully, folks from businesses and organizations such as Equal Exchange and Rainforest Alliance are helping us reach these farmers.

Let's look at the details of the coffee situation. First, a study conducted for the Consumer's Choice Council in October 1999, "Sustainable Coffee at the Crossroads," began with the following description of the coffee crisis: "Coffee is steeped in a number of social and environmental problems, including: massive deforestation caused by the transition from shade to sun coffee; degradation of soils and water sources; extremely low wages and poor working conditions for farmworkers on coffee estates; low prices paid to growers by commercial middlemen; and inequitable international distribution of the fruits of the gourmet coffee boom."[11]

As with so many commodities, skyrocketing production of coffee is running roughshod on the environment and on those who grow it. But, unlike most tropical crops, shade-grown coffee can truly coexist with the multitude of flora, fauna and multi-species ecosystems within a rainforest canopy. The Rainforest Alliance newsletter reported that, unfortunately, "Traditional coffee farms are rapidly undergoing 'technification' to the modern, agrochemical intensive, 'full-sun' management system that hosts little or no biodiversity."[12]

And just like some commodities in the US, with all the supposed "efficiency" inputs of pesticides and the like, coffee can cost more to produce than the market pays. As a result, the environmental degradation continues unabated. In the

> **Shopping tip**
>
> "Shade-grown coffee can truly coexist with the multitude of flora, fauna and multi-species ecosystems within a rainforest canopy."

introduction of her new book, *Coffee with Pleasure: Just Java and World Trade*, Laurie Waridel explains, "Because current coffee prices do not even cover the basic cost of production, many farmers are looking for more lucrative uses for their land. Some peasants are cutting down the forest, selling their wood and cheaply renting their land to large livestock owners. In other areas, coffee plantations are being turned into sugarcane fields."[13]

So prices are lower than ever. "How can this be?," you ask. Okay, so those Maxwell House cans do seem to be perpetually on sale, but gourmet coffees can still garner a good deal of a week's grocery budget. It is outrageous, as Waridel writes, that "middlemen are paying peasants in Mexico around 44¢ for a kilogram of coffee that will cost North American or European consumers at least $8 and sometimes as much as $30."[14] One of the reasons for this disparity is the number of middlemen along the way. Many farm families get cash loans with interest rates of 20 percent or more from the "coyotes," a word used to describe these dealers. Then, of course, they are beholden to sell their harvest to that same coyote who offers rock-bottom prices. Though cooperatives offer a slightly better alternative, most farmers cannot wait and sell their entire crop through cooperatives — they need some cash to feed their families out of season. So, off they go to the coyote for a short-term but ultimately long-effecting loan. A graphic depiction of the traditional coffee route is available on the website of a Canadian group encouraging change, Equiterre. They are in the midst of conducting "A Just Coffee" campaign, promoting fair trade through the coffee example. Their website describes their work: "A team of volunteers and employees organize a variety of public-information activities and encourage business owners to make Fair Trade coffee more accessible." Check out their website **<www.equiterre.qc.ca>** for more information on the subject.

There are now a handful of wonderful groups, and many of them have been working on kicking out a few of the profiteers, from bean to brew. Some work with cooperatives of farmers, while others encourage commitment to shade-grown production methods.

Three major types of efforts appear to be going on in the industry to help turn around the crisis, along with a handful of other creative enterprises. The three biggies you will find in many supermarkets (and if you don't, request them!) are: organic, shade-grown, and Fair Trade.

Shopping tip

"Three major types of efforts appear to be going on in the industry to help turn around the crisis: organic, shade-grown, and Fair Trade."

WEBSITE

But first a little background on coffee to help recognize the choices, because you won't find these labels on your typical can of coffee. Many of the canned coffees in the grocery store are either industrial or just-barely-specialty coffees of lower grades. Most of these are the bean Robusta, a commercial variety of pretty poor taste, most of which comes from Vietnam. (Similar to China's expanding apple production, Vietnam has increased production of Robusta exponentially in recent years.) The superior quality coffee beans, Arabica, need a bit more tender loving care. For years, coffee in cans used to come as approximately 70 percent Arabica. Now with rock-bottom prices for the Robusta, the percentage has switched.

Now to the three initiatives: organic, shade-grown and Fair Trade. Organic coffee is something we can understand: beans grown without the use of pesticides or inorganic fertilizers. Currently, according to a paper prepared for the Consumer's Choice Council, there are "250,000 hectares of certified organic and an estimated 3–4 million acres of uncertified organic coffee worldwide. Estimated US retail sales were $150 million in 1998, which is 3–5 percent of specialty coffee industry."[15] Although we consumers are more familiar with the term "organic" and may be more likely to buy it over the other terms we don't understand, there are some tricky issues with certified organic coffee. Many of the smallest farmers already use organic methods, but cannot afford the cost of certification. As reported in the *Ottawa Citizen*, "Most of them already farm organically and under shade, because they can't afford chemical fertilizer and insecticide. To be certified organic takes three years and a minimum $6,000 to $7,000 US, depending who is doing the certifying"[16] Purchasing organic coffee *does*, however, send the message that northern drinkers want pesticide-free coffee, and in turn may help reverse the mad rush to sun-grown industrial methods. We must speak louder for it, however. At this point, the message is not getting far enough back into the chain of custody. According to one coyote, "All the coffee gets lumped here. Organic coffee has been fashionable but it is an insignificant part of the market and really, farmers around here have been organic for many years. It doesn't help if you don't have a market to sell to."[17]

Next is shade-grown. Arabica grows best under shade, with only two hours of direct sunlight per day. For this reason, keeping the forest intact instead of cutting it

> **Shopping tip**
>
> *"Purchasing organic coffee does, however, send the message that northern drinkers want pesticide free coffee, and in turn may help reverse the mad rush to sun-grown industrial methods."*

down for the direct sun–pesticide version or even the farmer-constructed shade trellis version is preferable. "A study by the Smithsonian Institution in Washington found that destruction of forests to make way for coffee plantations in Central and South America has reduced the population of some migrating birds — Baltimore orioles included — by almost half.[18]" It sounds like an update on *Silent Spring* to me. This time we aren't destroying birds' eggshells with pesticides, we are taking away their homes. Is this what was meant by having "dominion" over the rest of the species? I just think a little more care was expected.

The last of the three labeling programs is Fair Trade. This concept was first practiced in the US by Equal Exchange, a worker-owned cooperative formed in 1986 to "buy coffee directly, and only, from democratically organized small farmer organizations in accordance with internationally recognized fair trade standards." As the Netherlands had been the world pioneer in Fair Trade, Equal Exchange adopted the Dutch standards in 1991. Today, 100 percent of the exchange's coffee is fairly traded. The 2001 premium to growers (the extra paid above market prices) was estimated at nearly a million dollars, approximately 12 percent of their total annual revenue. In that year, they imported 1,600,000 pounds of green coffee directly from 17 Fair Trade-registered co-ops in ten countries.

> ## Shopping tip
>
> *"The basic principle of Fair Trade coffee is that growers will receive a minimum of $1.26 per pound of coffee, no matter what the market brings."*

The basic principle of Fair Trade coffee is that growers will receive a minimum of $1.26 per pound of coffee, no matter what the market brings. While many growers are receiving the lowest prices in 100 years (around 63¢ per pound), Fair Trade growers maintain their $1.26, period.

In the mid 1990s, a handful of non-profit organizations were working to bring a national third-party certifier of Fair Trade coffee to the country. TransFair was first incorporated as its own non-profit organization in 1996, housed under the Institute of Agriculture and Trade Policy (IATP) in Minneapolis. In 1998, TransFair relocated to Oakland, California, and began operations (certification and market development for Fair Trade coffee). There are 17 Fair Trade certifications around the world under Fair Trade Labelling Organisations-International (FLO-International). Fair TradeMark Canada applied its TransFair logo to 200,000 pounds of beans in 1999. Cdn $3.90 per kilo of Arabica coffee is the minimum price paid.

Thankfully, it is not just a handful of large farmers who receive the lion's share of the premiums, as is the case in the US for government subsidies. Fair Trade also means small cooperatives, usually worker-owned and democratically run. In some cases, technical support and even solid loan programs to improve the community are provided by buyers.

TransFair USA reports accelerated increases in volume of Fair Trade coffee certified each year since its inception. In 1999, 2 million pounds were certified, and in 2001, they anticipated a total of 7 million pounds. More than 100 coffee companies now sell one or more coffees certified by TransFair USA. Consumers can find them by looking for Transfair's Fair Trade Certified label in their local food co-ops, natural food stores, and increasingly, mainstream outlets such as Starbucks, Trader Joe's, and Safeway and other supermarket chains. Again, much of the Fair Trade coffee success will depend on our willingness to purchase it. TransFair, Equal Exchange, and a growing number of non-profit organizations have consumer education efforts under way to get more retailers to carry Fair Trade coffee and ensure that it sells well once it is on the shelves. To find out which coffee companies and retailers carry Fair Trade Certified coffees, visit TransFair's website, **<www.transfairusa.org>**. A real coup for Fair Trade coffee resulted in Starbucks' willingness to carry the certified product in April 2000. Apparently it did not come easily. After nearly a year of concerted efforts by Global Exchange, a San Francisco-based human rights organization, Starbucks finally agreed.

More recently, Starbucks has announced new coffee purchasing guidelines, this time through pioneering efforts with the Center for Environmental Leadership in Business, an arm of Conservation International. The purchasing guidelines are based on the recently published *Conservation Principles for Coffee Production*, developed by the Consumer's Choice Council, Conservation International, the Rainforest Alliance, and the Smithsonian Migratory Bird Center.

It certainly is a step in the right direction. The principles of the new Starbucks guidelines seem inclusive, but they are also open to interpretation. Sustainable livelihoods, ecosystem and wildlife conservation, soil conservation, water conservation and protection, energy conservation, waste management, and pest and disease management are the guidelines' categories, with specific applications expected under each. As with any certification program, third-party verification (from someone outside the process) will ensure the rules are followed.

Principles like these need to be seemingly exhaustive, because coffee-growing is complicated. To avoid falling into many of the traps we have discussed in earlier chapters, it is important to take the long view. "Buying certified coffee is not a short-term solution; it is a complex and long-term solution to putting the power of the marketplace back in our hands," says Christopher London of the Consumer's Choice Council. "As consumers of coffee, we have the power to make the market work for us, to make it reflect our needs and concerns."[19]

Chocolate, bananas, citrus, and more and more

The other treats we indulge in from overseas have much the same story — particularly chocolate. Cocoa beans are grown very much like coffee, most naturally under shade. As prices plummet, cocoa growers look to the fastest, cheapest alternative: cut down those trees and add pesticides, resulting in larger harvests but very weak plants. Thanks to a British filmmaker's documentary, "Slavery," about the Ivory Coast, where 40 percent of the world's cocoa is produced, some serious ethical considerations about child labor were brought into question. Again, the answer is certified products. If your favorite non-organic chocolate bars are simply impossible to set aside, send the message to the company that you have had enough of unacceptable environmental and socially unjust agricultural practices.

I would like to describe my personal experience with bananas. Faced with children who love bananas (I don't care for them that much, especially since I found out how much more potassium is in potatoes than in bananas!), but the children love them, and they are an easy lunchbox addition. They also add great taste to pancakes. Over the years, I had heard about Chiquita working with the Rainforest Alliance. As it turns out, they have worked hard over the past ten years to improve their environmental growing practices. The Rainforest Alliance describes its environmental achievements: "100 percent of company-owned farms in Latin America have achieved certification; more than 71,000 acres covering 127 farms are certified; certification covers 90 percent of Chiquita's banana volume to Europe and two thirds to North America; dramatic agrochemical reductions including up to 80 percent lower use of herbicides; and more than 2,225 acres have been reforested with native trees."[20]

Knowing that Chiquita is a big multinational corporation, I was instinctively reticent. I had also heard about the hullabaloo at the *Cincinnati Enquirer* a few years ago (1998) when a reporter was fired for stealing personal messages for a story he was doing on Chiquita's bad practices. The content of his reports, however, was not called into question. I was in a quandary. So I went to the Internet and began my search. After reviewing a variety of documents, I headed to <**www.responsibleshopper.org**>, a website managed by Working Assets and Co-op America, providing ratings of companies by the Council on Economic Priorities. They shared the good news and the bad about Chiquita and gave the company overall good ratings.

Today I prefer to buy organic first, then Chiquita bananas ahead of other multinationals, primarily because of their involvement with the Rainforest Alliance, an organization I respect. But I had to do more research to feel okay about the decision. It isn't perfect, and it may not last. I may learn of a small banana grower doing all sorts of wonderful things, and I'll switch. Choosing eco-foods isn't always easy, but it certainly is good for the Earth and for us all.

> **Shopping tip**
>
> *"Today I prefer to buy organic first, then Chiquita bananas ahead of other multinationals, primarily because of their involvement with the Rainforest Alliance, an organization I respect."*

It would be wonderful if our growing interest in overseas foodstuffs was limited to the truly unusual, but it is not. According to the *FDA Consumer*, "The estimated value of food imports in 1998 hit $32 billion, a new US record. Moreover, food imports exceeded exports in 1998 by $2.6 billion, the first US agricultural trade deficit since 1991."[21]

We want what they have, or at least we are encouraged to do so. All sorts of corporate pressures exist to fill our markets with a cornucopia of international foodstuffs.

NAFTA, GATT, and world trade

NAFTA

Let's pursue a little history lesson in world trade, starting on our own continent with the North American Free Trade Agreement (NAFTA.) Enacted in 1994, the purpose of NAFTA was to open borders between Mexico, the US, and Canada, providing access to new markets and relief from economic hardship. Unfortunately, there are real questions about NAFTA and if it has provided any relief.

Mexico seems to have suffered the most. According to a report in *Public Citizen*, "Before NAFTA, two to three million Mexican peasant farmers were growing (at subsistence-level) corn ... Remarkably, these small farmers produced a surplus each year that supplied about 40 percent of Mexico's domestic commercial corn market, enough to keep the nation close to food sufficiency. By 1996, Mexico had lost more than half its small farms. Thousands of tiny parcels that once grew corn for Mexicans had been consolidated and converted to the corporate production of berries, baby lettuce, mesclun mix, and asparagus for export. The domestic consumption of corn and other basic food had dropped by 29 percent." How did this happen? The US introduced cheap corn into Mexico, lowering the price the small farmers received and making it virtually impossible to stay in business. This is sometimes referred to as "dumping." In the meantime, some large US corporations have moved across the southern border, where production is cheaper and easier. Again from *Public Citizen*: "For instance, a quantity of the huge new NAFTA flood of tomatoes and peppers are coming from transnational agribusinesses which relocated to Mexico to access $3.60/day rural labor, exploit the use of pesticides banned in the US and enjoy unlimited duty-free access back into the US consumer market."[22]

You would think if Mexico fared so poorly, the US and Canada must have done well. To the contrary, it seems no one (except maybe big business) has done well with this agreement. It appears imports to the US outpaced exports to Mexico and Canada. We know that US farmers have found no relief since the agreement's inception, with farmers going out of business and prices falling to below production costs.

Canada apparently has received a substantial increase in export dollars. Eighty-five percent of Canada's exports go to its southern neighbor.[23] Similar to the Mexican corn issue, inexpensive tomatoes seem to be crisscrossing borders, Canadian greenhouse tomatoes into the US and US field tomatoes into Canada. For both players, commodity prices have been forced down by negotiations within the expanded market.

One of the most surprising results of NAFTA has been the US government's interest in expanding the agreement to include South American countries in the Free Trade Area of the Americas. Further, the Bush administration wants a faster, "more efficient" process of negotiating trade with the new Fast Track trade authority. This would basically take away negotiating power from Congress and turn it over to the administration. It seems to me that these agreements might need *more* dialogue with greater input for positive solutions … not *less*.

GATT and the WTO

In 1948, 23 countries drew up the General Agreement on Tariffs and Trade (GATT) following a conference held the previous year in Geneva. The original intention of the conference was to consider a draft charter for an International Trade Organization (which did not happen for many more years).

The GATT's basic premise is that participating members would accord each other "non-discriminatory, most favored nation treatment" (meaning you will treat everyone the same as you would treat your most favored trading partner) with respect to tariffs, with no quantitative restrictions on imports or exports. The GATT also contained a long list of rules and regulations and other provisions that were picked up along the way in various rounds of negotiations. The Uruguay Round, ending in 1994, created the World Trade Organization (WTO), a legal institution — the rulemaster of international trade.

Some of the rules concern me. For example, one says all nations must subvert their own laws to abide by world trade. An example of potential ramifications comes from the 1995 New York state budget where, buried in legislative-ese, was a list of laws to be eliminated because they conflicted with WTO rules, including one that favored the purchase of New York state-produced food.[24] Thankfully, those laws were not eliminated, but imagine not being able to give preference to your own state's produce?!

Another thing that bothers me about the WTO's governing capacity is the secrecy of its documents and proceedings. Everything is handled in confidence, with little opportunity to dispute. Again, with the stakes as high and the influence as great as they are, it would seem more eyes, more positive thinking, and more input would be appropriate. It seems the fear is that we, the consumers, might learn something ... about how little attention is being paid to our environment, about how much of our tax dollars goes to subsidize the corporate dumping of crops in other countries, where our brothers and sisters there fight to feed their families. We might learn that the profiteers are fundamentally skewing best practices.

Wendell Berry says it clearly: "Consumers who feel a prompting toward land stewardship find that in this economy they can have no stewardly practice. To be a consumer in the total economy, one must agree to be totally ignorant, totally passive, and totally dependent on distant supplies and self-interested suppliers."[25]

But in naiveté, I believe in people, the power of our individual choices, and our ability to say "No more!" According to Maude Barlow, national chairperson of the Council of Canadians and a director with the International Forum on Globalization, "Free trade is the problem. Fair trade is the solution. Currently world trade is dominated by the ideology of economic globalization — the creation of a single global economy with universal rules set by big business for big business in which a seamless global consumer market operates on free-market principles, unfettered by domestic or international laws or standards. This system of trade is controlled by a handful of transnational corporations operating outside any domestic law or any international rules except business-friendly trade agreements. And it is creating deep and entrenched inequalities in its wake."[26]

> "We can buy Fair Trade coffee. We can buy locally grown foods. We can learn about the problems and share the solutions with our friends. Today, right now, right here in this moment, we can be the solution."

We can buy Fair Trade coffee. We can buy locally grown foods. We can do the research to find out which brand of bananas is the best for today. We can write our senators and our congressmen. We can learn about the problems and share the solutions with our friends. Today, right now, right here in this moment, we can be the solution. Just by reading this, you are participating in changing the world.

9

Conveyor Belt Food

FROM FIELD TO FORK, PROCESSING (moving food from a fresh whole product to a preserved and sometimes prepared product) takes most of your food dollar and adds a lot of extra … stuff. Maybe our grandmothers had the time to pull up fresh carrots, onions, and herbs for the day's soup broth, mill the grain and knead the dough for the dinner's bread loaf, or bake a backyard berry pie for dessert, but I certainly don't! I wish I did, and yet …

According to Rachel Laudan, writing for the magazine *Gastronomica*, Grandma wasn't so happy with her role of chief cook and bottle washer. "Churning butter and skinning and cleaning hares, without the option of picking up the phone for a pizza if something goes wrong is unremitting, unforgiving toil."[1] Laudan would call me a culinary Luddite, looking back through food history with rose-colored glasses. I see only the alone time Grandma got while calmly and quietly humming her way through meal preparation, a luxury I often fantasize about. But would I be willing to let go of writing a book or working with growers to help bring environmental products to market? Would I be willing to do nothing but cook?

I just mentioned to my husband that this month would probably bring lots of take-out Chinese to our table, considering the deadline I am trying to meet. And what a luxury that is. The final decision for tonight, instead, was a quick pasta dish: frozen raviolis with some sauce I will whip up using organic canned tomatoes, fresh spices, and grated Parmesan. Grandma is not around to make the fresh pasta or can the tomatoes or even grate the cheese. I am depending on our culture of processed foods to bring a fast feast to my family. Manufacturers have taken over Grandma's role, but they don't have as much concern for our health and well being as she did.

How does it add up?

So how involved are those manufacturers? If it costs 10¢ to grow enough peaches to fill a can, why does the can cost almost a dollar? In essence, the other 90¢ goes to marketing: transportation, food processing, and packaging.

With our hard-earned dollars, it seems we prefer to buy foods that have been handled. In 1973, 21¢ of every food dollar was spent on manufactured foods; this increased to 41¢ in 1987, and now it's at 90¢.[2] We may like our peaches fresh, but more often we buy them processed.

> "In 1973, 21¢ of every food dollar was spent on manufactured foods; this increased to 41¢ in 1987, and now it's at 90¢.[2] We may like our peaches fresh, but more often we buy them processed."

What do they do to those peaches? Just as in Grandma's day, peaches need syrup when canned. Okay. But first they need to be peeled and pitted, then cooked, put into cans, sealed, labeled, put into packages, and put onto trucks. Lots of time and energy, additives, and big equipment mean a big bill. Food processing is big business. According to the Economic Research Service of the USDA, more than 26,000 food processing plants employ 1.47 million workers, just over 1 percent of all US employment. Most of these plants are small; only 4 percent have 100 or more employees, but these account for 80 percent of the value added in food processing. We have talked about the concentration and multinational power associated with many of these processing plants. In 1992, sales of processed foods in the US amounted to almost $406 billion, the fifth largest sector of the US economy.[3]

It is no big surprise that processing has become such a huge percentage of our food dollar. We like the convenience. We like our food to stay fresh longer. We like the breadth of choice. Here we go again, all about the consumer and what we want. We certainly send signals, even if they are not our well-thought-out decisions.

We know the largest sector of the processing world is meat manufacturing. We like meat, carnivores that we humans are, but we don't want to see meat whole. The days of cooking a whole pig over a pit are dwindling. Most of our meat comes in packages. Chicken seems more readily available in parts — thighs, breasts, and drumsticks — than as whole birds. The meat industry is scary. The big processors control the process, from the way animals are raised to the way they are packaged. Along with the antibiotics they serve to our animals, what can they be adding when they process the meat? How does meat have such a long shelf life these days?

Processors are allowed to use all sorts of salts, binders, fillers, anti-caking agents, and gelling agents. They are also allowed to add colors! We might want to take a closer look at labels. What do they put in our foodstuffs?

Nutrition Lesson No. 2

Back to peaches as an example. The processor adds sugar and takes away the skins, the part of the fruit nutritionists tell us is packed with good-for-us things like pectin and unusual nutrients. We can often see what is being removed, but it is very difficult to see what has been added. Welcome to the world of food additives.

> "We can often see what is being removed, but it is very difficult to see what has been added. Welcome to the world of food additives."

According to the Food and Drug Administration, "In its broadest sense, a food additive is any substance added to food. Legally, the term refers to 'any substance the intended use of which results or may reasonably be expected to result — directly or indirectly — in its becoming a component or otherwise affecting the characteristics of any food.' This definition includes any substance used in the production, processing, treatment, packaging, transportation or storage of food."[4]

Additives range from colorings to preservatives. It is hard enough to keep on top of names like ibuprofen and acetaminophen (common pain relievers); imagine trying to rattle off names like methyl cellulose or disodium guanylate — the first is a tricky fiber our kidneys may have trouble handling, and the latter is relatively safe unless you are suffering from gout. So get out your notebooks and pens. We have 300 or so of the top additives to learn.

Our brains can take only so much. So instead, we trust our governments to keep us safe from anything too serious. How do they do this? In the US, the basic law that governs food additives is the Federal Food, Drug, and Cosmetic (FD&C) Act of 1938, amended in 1958, to require FDA approval of additives prior to their inclusion in food. It also requires the manufacturer to prove an additive's safety.

To quote the Food and Drug Administration again:

The Food Additives Amendment exempted two groups of substances from the food additive regulation process. All substances that FDA or the US Department of Agriculture (USDA) had determined were safe for use in specific food prior to the 1958 amendment were designated as prior-sanctioned substances. Examples of prior-sanctioned substances are sodium nitrite and potassium nitrite, used to preserve luncheon meats.

A second category of substances excluded from the food additive regulation process are generally recognized as safe, or GRAS, substances. GRAS substances are those whose use is generally recognized by experts as safe, based on their extensive history of use in food before 1958, or based on published scientific evidence. Salt, sugar, spices, vitamins, and monosodium glutamate are classified as GRAS substances, along with several hundred other substances.

In 1960, Congress passed the Color Additives Amendments governing the use of colors. In contrast to food additives, colors in use before the legislation were allowed continuous use only if they underwent further testing to confirm their safety. Of the original 200 provisionally listed color additives, 90 have been listed as safe, and the remainder have either been removed from use by FDA or withdrawn by industry.

Both the Food Additives and Color Additives Amendments include a provision (known as the Delany Clause) which prohibits the approval of an additive if it is found to cause cancer in humans or animals. Regulations known as Good Manufacturing Practices (GMP) limit the amount of food and color additives used in foods. Manufacturers use only the amount of an additive necessary to achieve the desired effect.[5]

In 1985, the FDA began the Adverse Reactions Monitoring System, which reacts to consumers' or doctors' complaints by logging issues into a database and following up on recurring problems. Many of the complaints to date have been about the sugar substitute aspartame.

In Canada, regulation is under the Canadian Food and Drugs Act and carried out by Health Canada. One of the best books published on the subject of food additives is *Hard to Swallow: The Truth About Food Additives*, with a foreword by Dr. Rose Hume Hall, a professor emeritus at McMaster University in Canada. It prints out sections of the Food and Drugs Act, highlights certain suspicious additives and suspect language, and provides authors' notes throughout the legal text. In addition, Dr. Hall shares her brief and frustrating experience with the political side of food additives in the foreword, a real eye-opener about the regulatory arena. The real highlight of the book is an alphabetical guide to 300 food additives. If you are interested in learning more about the possible dangers of food additives, this is a great book.

Another source of information is the Center for Science in the Public Interest website, **<www.cspinet.org>**. Its "Chemical Cuisine: CSPI's Guide to Food Additives" provides an easy-to-use listing of additives with icons indicating the following:

WEBSITE

• Safe. The additive appears to be safe.
• Cut back on this. Not toxic, but large amounts may be unsafe or promote bad nutrition.
• Caution. May pose a risk and needs to be better tested. Try to avoid.
• Certain people should avoid these additives.
• Everyone should avoid. Unsafe in amounts consumed or is very poorly tested and not worth any risk.

The list is only 73 items long, with the following falling into the "avoid" category: Acesulfame-K, artificial colorings, aspartame, BHA and BHT, caffeine, monosodium glutamate, nitrite and nitrate, Olestra, potassium bromate, saccharin, and sulfites. The website contains full descriptions of each of these, their current health implications, and in what foods they are most often found. This is a list I can comprehend and may even be able to retain.

If it still seems like too much to try to remember, CSPI suggests, "A simple general rule about additives is to avoid sodium nitrite, saccharin, caffeine, Olestra, Acesulfame-K, and artificial coloring. Not only are they among the most questionable additives, but they are used primarily in foods of low nutritional value. Also, don't forget the two most familiar additives: sugar and salt. They may pose the greatest risk because we consume so much of them."[6]

Beyond additives, what else do the manufacturers do to our food? Irradiation is a new one, a danger or a

> ## Shopping tip
>
> *"A simple general rule about additives is to avoid sodium nitrite, saccharin, caffeine, Olestra, Acesulfame-K, and artificial coloring. Also, don't forget the two most familiar additives: sugar and salt."*

safeguard, depending on how you look at it. It is a process of using radiation to kill microorganisms or bacteria in our foodstuff. With the onslaught of new foodborne diseases caused by *E. coli* or salmonella, the idea of ridding our food of any potential pathogens is welcomed by some. However, the idea of using radiation on anything gives pause to others, including myself.

The normal processing of foods results in the development of "free radicals." Some research shows that irradiation creates many times the normal number. The problem with this is that free radicals have been found to be cancer-causing. As reported in the *International Journal of Health Services,* "A wide range of independent studies prior to 1986 clearly identified mutagenic and carcinogenic radiolytic products (the combination of free radicals and other compounds) in irradiated food, and confirmed evidence of genetic toxicity in tests on irradiated food."[7] In addition, food irradiation results in major losses of micronutrients, particularly vitamins A, C, E, and the B complex."[8]

The organic community has fought to prohibit the use of irradiation as part of the national standards and has won. If knowledgeable people are concerned enough about this process to fight for clarification in the national organic standards, I believe I should not purchase foods that have been irradiated. This is an example of my trusting a group's recommendations when my ability to clarify the research is limited. Sometimes I simply need to make today's eco-foods choices based on the data I have and the viewpoints of those I trust.

> "The organic community has fought to prohibit the use of irradiation as part of the national standards and has won. If knowledgeable people are concerned enough about this process to fight for clarification in the national organic standards, I believe I should not purchase foods that have been irradiated."

Currently the majority of the irradiation has been within the meat industry. Speaking directly of sanitation in feedlot pens (where most animals raised for meat are kept), Dr. Samuel Epstein, professor emeritus of environmental medicine and chairman of the Cancer Prevention Coalition, University of Illinois School of Public Health, says, "The focus of the radiation and agribusiness industries is directed to the highly lucrative cleanup of contaminated food rather than to preventing contamination at its source."

Well, chalk it up as another item to look for on labels. You may not find the term "irradiation" anymore. Those in the industry have developed a much nicer, less frightening term: electronic pasteurization. However, the print size used to identify irradiation can be as small as the size used for the ingredients. You might consider taking a magnifying glass to the store, or you could look for the attractive and non-disturbing radura icon which looks like a broken green circle with a stylized flower inside.

An end to this story

There can be an end to this story when we make choices for the health of our Earth and for ourselves. How much power do we give away when we buy products that have been processed in ways we don't totally trust? How many times have we purchased food or drinks, knowing they contain dyes, aspartame, or Olestra? If you are like me, plenty. We can, however, choose foods that have been manufactured appropriately. According to Rachel Laudan, "Far from fleeing them, we should be clamoring for more high-quality industrial foods."[9]

Although one alternative is to seek out more packaged goods that are labeled as having no additives, my preferred solution is to put up our own food with full knowledge of what we used in the processing. This doesn't mean staying up until midnight over a hot stove in August. It could be as simple as popping some blueberries in the freezer or turning tomatoes into salsa. With the advent of food processors, it may be a lot easier than we think. Publications such as the *Ball Blue Book* and *Putting Food By* make it easier for amateur at-home processors to enter the world of manufacturing, even if it is just for our own larder. Every time I buy fresh sweet corn from the roadside stands in the summer, I buy a dozen. My family will usually eat six or seven, and I remove the corn from the rest of the ears and bag it up for the freezer.

> "my preferred solution is to put up our own food with full knowledge of what we used in the processing. It could be as simple as popping some blueberries in the freezer or turning tomatoes into salsa."

Another quick-freeze item is pesto. By early September, I have seven or eight ice-cube trays full of the basil sauce. That way, in a pinch, I can pop out as many cubes as there are people to feed that night. Granted, most of us don't have the time to put up a significant percentage of our winter diet, but every little bit helps. If you are considering this option, it might be wise to review the books and materials available on proper storage and handling as a safety precaution.

We can also buy more fresh, whole foods. Until I found out how easy it is to use a whole, fresh pumpkin for making pies, I, too, succumbed to the canned version.

Now when my mother comes to visit, she arrives with a pumpkin under her arm and a plea in her heart. It does taste better, and who knows what chemicals my family avoids? I suppose I could not do this without the resources of our community-supported farm, farmers' markets, or roadside stands and the immediate presence of whole foods. Lured by the convenience of packaged goods, it is often a difficult decision to make. On the other hand, knowing the risks we take with artificially colored and flavored foods, it is good to know we still have a choice.

10

Bio(tech) Hazards

THEY CALL THEM "FRANKENFOODS" BECAUSE THEY START IN THE LAB AND COME
OUT ... well, we have yet to find out. And surveys say if we can get away with
it, we would rather not know anything about them. They're out there, in 70 percent
of our foods. So let's take the plunge into the world of biotech together.

I must tell the truth. This subject has seriously intimidated me over the years. I
wanted to avoid it altogether, it seemed so big and overwhelming. The name is even
frightening: biotechnology. How would I understand all the issues, or even what it
is? I am not terribly surprised by the recent Rutgers University's Food Policy
Institute poll that said, "Only four in 10 respondents in a survey conducted by the
university's Food Policy Institute said they are aware that genetically modified foods
are sold at their local market, and more than two-thirds said they have never had a
conversation about biotechnology."[1] Initially, I had hoped to give more in-depth
information about both sides of the biotechnology issue, but after reading,
discussing, and digesting more than my share (or at least I think so — products
containing GMOs are not allowed to be labeled as such), I must admit before you
even begin to read, this is not an unbiased review. I have tried to see the positive, but
I just can't find it. I have had my share of corporate public relations jobs, but this one
I certainly would not be able to do. On the other side, I wouldn't call myself a
Luddite. I am just a working mom who wants to do the right thing at home and for

the Earth. For this reason, this chapter may have more authoritative quotes than you have seen from me so far. So, opinionated as it is, here goes … my take on biotech.

It may have started with a few peas, but it took a real leap

Advocates of biotech like to say that Gregor Mendel started the whole shebang years ago when he decided to crossbreed a few pea plants. Hybridization — crossing two similar plants to achieve characteristics of both parents — took off. Over the years, plant breeding evolved into a sophisticated method of encouraging or limiting certain genetic traits in a plant. These traits helped farmers cope with environmental conditions. Many of the new varieties were drought resistant, or naturally pest- or disease-resistant; some made more beautiful flowers than ever seen before; others had thicker stems to withstand winds; and most produced greater yields.

Even though advocates do like to suggest biotech is simply an extension of something we have been doing for years, from what I can see, genetic engineering is quite different. There is a source to understand the difference. A wonderful PBS/Nova website, **<www.pbs.org/wgbh/harvest/engineer/>**, actually takes you through the steps of each method of modification, the classical crossbreeding and the genetically engineered. In the pathway "Engineer a Crop," you are asked to make the various decisions entailed in genetically modifying an organism. It is a very helpful tool.

As I understand it, crossbreeding mates two like species/varieties to get a result with favorable qualities. With genetic engineering, scientists actually remove a specific gene from one thing and physically add it to the other thing. The real difference seems to be in the ability to mate unlike objects, impossible in classical breeding. I like long-time biotech opponent Jeremy Rifkin's simple explanation in an interview with Nova: "In classical breeding, you can cross close relatives… You can, for example, cross various wheat strains and corn strains, etc…. You can cross a donkey and a horse in classical breeding — they're very close relatives — and you can get a mule. But you can't cross a donkey and an apple tree in classical breeding. What the public needs to understand is that these new technologies, especially in recombinant DNA technology, allow scientists to bypass biological

> "What the public needs to understand is that these new technologies, especially in recombinant DNA technology, allow scientists to bypass biological boundaries altogether "

boundaries altogether... Crossing genetic information from one species to another is something we've never seen in 10,000 years of classical breeding."[2]

It appears genetic engineering is a whole different level of intervention. Many may consider commonplace breeding already on the fringe of what is within our purview to control and manipulate. But this new method seems to cross new boundaries. Michael Pollan, a writer whose work in this field I scramble to read, gave a poetic version of his experience of growing genetically engineered New Leaf potatoes (no longer on the market) in his *New York Times* article, "Playing God in the Garden.""Since distant species in nature cannot be crossed, the breeder's art has always run up against a natural limit of what a potato is willing, or able, to do. Nature, in effect, has exercised a kind of veto on what culture can do with a potato."[3]

Advocates of biotechnology seem to take a no-big-deal attitude that the whole process is fairly rudimentary, and that scientists have it under control. And, they suggest, we should simply put our trust in the lab work of those who brought us pesticides. Some scientists outside the corporate realm have a different message.

Brewster Kneen writes in his book *Farmageddon*, "As biologist Mae-Wan Ho puts it, 'To understand why genetic engineering biotechnology is so inherently hazardous, we have to appreciate the prodigious power of microbes to proliferate, the protein promiscuity of the genes they carry, and their ability to jump, spread, mutate and recombine.'"[4] This is probably why the mantra, "We just don't know enough," has become a central concern for those not sold on biotech.

The idea that we could once again be going down a slippery slope without enough knowledge is frightening. Dr. John Fagan, a molecular biologist and former genetic engineer, compares it with our overzealous commitment to nuclear power years ago: "No one knew that nuclear power would bring us to the brink of annihilation or fill our planet with highly toxic radioactive waste. We were so excited by the power of a new discovery that we leapt ahead blindly, and without caution. Today the situation with genetic engineering is perhaps even more grave because this technology acts on the very blueprint of life itself."[5]

Putting one thing into another thing. How hard can it be to identify the possibilities? If you understand all the possibilities for A and all the possibilities for B and add them, then consider all the possibilities for A+B, you would think that would do it. But it doesn't, of course, because the organisms aren't stagnant and reliable, they are alive. They have behaviors that, in combination, go far beyond anything we might consider as A+B. Let's let Jeremy Rifkin explain this concept: "When you introduce a genetically modified organism into the environment, it's not like introducing a chemical product, or even a nuclear product. Remember, genetically modified products are alive. So at the get-go, they're inherently more unpredictable in terms of what they'll do once they're out into the environment. Secondly, GMOs reproduce. Chemical products don't do that. Third, they can mutate. Fourth, they can migrate and proliferate over wide regions. And fifth, you cannot easily recall them to the laboratory or clean them up."[6]

As astounding as it is to be able to put genes from one organism into another, it would be more astounding if we could actually know what will happen when we do. Martin Teitel says in his book, *Genetically Engineered Food: Changing the Nature of Nature*, "Moving a gene around may or may not produce the same result each time, because the gene and protein environment can be fantastically complex and infinitely variable. Most genetic engineering is a highly imprecise practice. Farmers and plant breeders know that genes are mutable, and many factors, including the environment, play a major role in the expression or adaptation of a gene or genetic trait."[7] So what might make sense in a fairly controlled environment on a test field in temperate northern California may not make any sense in a recently clearcut rainforest in a small tropical country.

Michael Pollan asked Harvard University geneticist Richard Lewontin for a metaphor for biotechnology: "'An ecosystem,' he offered. 'You can always intervene and change something in it, but there's no way of knowing what all the downstream effects will be or how it might affect the environment. We have such a miserably poor understanding of how the organism develops from its DNA that I would be surprised if we don't get one rude shock after another.'"[8] So the concept of A+B is way off. You would have to multiply this sum by all the environments and all the potential weather conditions and all the variables of time plus a few other multipliers I can't even guess. Do you think the scientists or academics contracted by those multinationals anticipate all the variables?

Remember, we are talking about the same players who brought us the chemicals on our fields that we are now trying to avoid. They used to be called chemical companies. Today they are known as "life science" companies.

On "Harvest of Fear," a program aired on PBS on April 24, 2001, the narrator reminds us, "In 1947, *Time* magazine carried an advertisement claiming that DDT was good for people, homes, and farms. It took 20 years before scientists realized how dangerous it was." Jane Rissler from the Union of Concerned Scientists replies, "So if you just replace that with '*Biotechnology* is good for me' see, these same people who once told us that pesticides were good for us are now saying, 'Well, those pesticides, they're dangerous. But you take these biotech products. They're much safer."[9] And biotech is supposed to be a big solution to the pesticide problem?

So let's just take precautions!

If the big concern is that we don't have enough information, it would make sense to slow things down and take some precautions. Believe it or not, there is such a principle out there in the scientific community, referred to as the Precautionary Principle. Different than the traditional "risk assessment" approach, the principle suggests caution and foresight.

Brewster Kneen suggests, "There is a clear policy alternative to the subjective and inadequate process of risk assessment, and that is the 'precautionary principle,' which puts the burden of proof back where it belongs: on the proponents of 'plants with novel traits,' 'novel foods,' and all other forms of biotechnology that induce changes we barely comprehend."[10] Unfortunately, the concept is still controversial and application, although agreed to on an international level, has not taken off ... yet.

According to the Science and Environmental Health Network's *Precautionary Principle Handbook*, the concept of a precautionary principle was first brought beyond simple foresight as it applied to the environment in Germany in the 1970s. It was first introduced in 1984 at the First International Conference on Protection of the North Sea and incorporated into other international agreements since. In 1992, it was expressed in the Rio Declaration from the United Nations Conference on Environment and Development as follows: "In order to protect the environment, the precautionary approach shall be widely applied by States according to their capabilities. Where there are threats of serious or irreversible damage, lack of full scientific certainty shall not be used as a reason for postponing cost-effective measures to prevent environmental degradation."[11]

The US signed the Rio Declaration, and thus it is supposed to be adhering to the principle. However, it hasn't acted as such on a number of occasions, such as in trade disputes with the European Union. Angered that some EU countries were blocking the entrance of hormone-fed US beef by citing the precautionary principle, the US pulled punches with a trade tariff on specialty items, such as Roquefort cheese.

Watching the US vacillate on the application of the principle, Carolyn Raffensperger and her staff at the Science and Environmental Health Network brought together an international group of scientists, government officials, lawyers, and labor and grass-roots environmental activists in January 1998. From this session came the Wingspread Statement on the Precautionary Principle:

> While we realize that human activities may involve hazards, people must proceed more carefully than has been the case in recent history. Corporations, government entities, organizations, communities, scientists and other individuals must adopt a precautionary approach to all human endeavors.
>
> Therefore, it is necessary to implement the Precautionary Principle: When an activity raises threats of harm to human health or the environment, precautionary measures should be taken even if some cause and effect relationships are not fully established scientifically. In this context the proponent of an activity, rather than the public, should bear the burden of proof.
>
> The process of applying the Precautionary Principle must be open, informed and democratic and must include potentially affected parties. It must also involve an examination of the full range of alternatives, including no action.[12]

For years, science has remained committed to risk assessment, and even that hasn't gotten much attention, particularly in terms of resources. Today, the Precautionary Principle is a reality. For more information, pick up a copy of Carolyn Raffensperger's new book, *Protecting Public Health & the Environment: Implementing the Precautionary Principle.*

Would you care for some *Bacillus thuringiensis* (Bt) for lunch?

One item that appears to have bypassed the Precautionary Principle (again) is Bt corn. In a press release from the US Environmental Protection Agency dated October 16, 2001, Stephen L. Johnson, Assistant Administrator of EPA's Office of Prevention, Pesticides, and Toxic Substances said:

> Based on a comprehensive scientific review, corn genetically modified with *Bacillus thuringiensis* (Bt) has been approved for an additional seven years.
>
> *Bacillus thuringiensis* is a naturally-occurring soil bacterium that produces a protein toxic to certain insects, which has been used for many years to control insect pests ... Scientific studies and a history of successful use have demonstrated that Bt is not toxic to humans or other animals ...

Bt corn has been evaluated thoroughly by EPA, and we are confident that it does
not pose risks to human health or to the environment. Consumers should be assured
that these corn varieties show no signs of any adverse effects to human health.

Let's do a little background check on this product. First, remember when we first
chatted about GMOs in Chapter 2? We said that Bt corn was particularly destructive
to organic (and IPM) growers who are trying to use what few tools are available. Bt
is one of the least toxic naturally occurring (making it approved for organic)
chemicals out there. By inserting it into every single corn plant on a field, the
resulting resistance of corn borer caterpillars to the pesticide is sped up
significantly. What might have been a 30-year window becomes a three-year
window for successful results. Chuck Benbrook, a crop consultant and sustainable
agriculture advocate, estimates that, "up to 10,000 times as much Bt toxin is
produced in the crop as would have been used in typical external application — and
that's assuming a year in which the corn borer needed to be controlled at all."[13]

The manufacturer of the corn and the government have suggested alternatives to
reduce the resistance, such as building a refuge — a place where caterpillars can go
and eat as much non-GMO corn as their stomachs can hold. Then, the sellers surmise,
the resistant bugs will mate with the non-resistant bugs, thus slowing the process.

Some of you may be asking, "What about the butterflies?" Those of you who
landed on the Bt-modified-corn issue through the Monarch butterfly publicity may
be questioning the application of the Precautionary Principle here. The story
originally broke in 1999 in the journal *Nature*, when Cornell University scientist
John Losey reported that pollen from the Bt-pumped corn could poison the larvae
of Monarch butterflies. As a visual icon of nature for so many years, fear of the
Monarch's demise caused immediate alarm.

Timing is everything, it seems. Since approval for Bt corn was about to expire,
the EPA was required to take on a reassessment process before its renewal. With
environmental organizations hot on the trail, the EPA realized it would need further
study before a ruling could be made. Lincoln Brower's intriguing story in the
magazine *Orion* revealed the details of the resulting power struggle between
industry and their contracted scientists versus environmentalists and public-
supported scientists:

The industry's early responses to the Cornell paper were designed to cast doubt on
whether the scientists' laboratory findings were applicable to Monarch caterpillars

in the field. The agricultural industry's manipulation of the press was soon made even clearer. Several corporations, including the Monsanto Company, Novartis AG of Switzerland, and the Pioneer Hi-Bred of DuPont Company formed a soothingly named consortium, the Agricultural Biotechnology Stewardship Working Group (ABSWG). The ABSWG contacted university scientists and provided funding for studies that would address issues raised by the Cornell findings. US and Canadian scientists conducted a research program during the summer of 1999, the results of which were to be presented at a scientific symposium in Chicago on November 2, hosted by the ABSWG, and also attended by representatives of the EPA and the USDA. The avowed purpose of this symposium was for the scientists to present and discuss their findings, review their methodologies, and determine through consensus what information was inconclusive or missing.

Because of the hurried nature of their summer research, all of the meeting participants prefaced their scientific presentations with the caveat that their data and conclusions were preliminary. Some results indicated possible major impact, others suggested minor impact, and most agreed that the current research base could not resolve the problem.

At the meeting, Carol Yoon, a *New York Times* science journalist, made a stunning announcement: she had just received a fax from her editor, indicating that a media advisory had been released earlier in the day. The headline describing the still-in-progress meeting stated, "Scientific Symposium to Show No Harm to Monarch Butterfly." There was now no doubt that the symposium had been co-opted by the ABSWG, and that the press was being manipulated. Yoon's report exposing this fiasco, "No Consensus on the Effects of Engineering on Corn Crops," was published in the *Times* on November 4. The EPA's interim assessment of the risks and benefits ... stated, "The published preliminary monarch toxicity information is not sufficient to cause undue concern of harmful widespread effects to monarch butterflies at this time."

The following year, the summer 2000 research was presented to many of the same attendees. "The papers presented at this symposium reflected the complexities of the Bt corn issue. Working with different methodologies even in areas where their investigations overlapped, the scientists' findings were not easily compared."

In summary, despite the EPA's interim assessment, the overall database that had been assembled through November 2000 was not adequate to resolve whether Bt pollen is a significant detriment to the Monarch butterfly.[14]

For more information on the Monarch debate, check out the *Orion*-managed website, **<www.savethemonarchs.org>**.

So as of October 16, 2001, we have another seven years of Bt corn, and we have no conclusive research on its safety to Monarch butterflies. This does not sound precautionary to me. Putting the Monarch issue aside, what about the safety of Bt corn to us? I remember sharing this concern with a pro-GMO colleague (who, by the way, I truly respect), who said very clearly and definitively, "The Bt protein does not turn on in our system." I remember thinking that she must know a lot more than I do about this subject. It seems all I have are questions. She seemed to have the answers — at least one, anyway. Since then, I have tried to find out more about this, and apparently, scientifically, it is *not supposed* to turn on in our guts.

As Brewster Kneen suggests, "Theoretically, there is no problem because Bt is inactivated in acidic environments, such as the normal human gut — but not everyone is 'normal.' This has never been addressed because reductionist science, the corporate drive to get new products to market, and the regulatory agencies' simplistic conceptions of life see no reason to address it."[15]

You might have wondered why it was the EPA that was releasing its findings on Bt corn. It makes sense: Bt is a pesticide, so it would be under the purview of the EPA. However, it is also a food additive, so maybe the FDA should regulate it? No, it stays with the EPA, and subsequently the research on its effects as a component of food is limited. According to Miguel Altieri, writing for the Institute for Food and Development, "Recent evidence however shows that there are potential risks of eating such foods as the new proteins produced in such foods could: act themselves as allergens or toxins, alter the metabolism of the food producing plant or animal causing it to produce new allergens or toxins, or reduce its nutritional quality or value as in the case of herbicide resistant soybeans that contained less isoflavones, an important phytoestrogen present in soybeans, believed to protect women from a number of cancers."[16]

I particularly like the response from Margaret Mellon of the Union of Concerned Scientists in Michael Pollan's *New York Times* article. Remember, he grows Bt potatoes (no longer available) as a test. In the end, he is deciding if it is safe to eat them. He calls Mellon, a molecular biologist, for advice. "She couldn't offer any hard scientific evidence that my New Leafs [potatoes] were unsafe, though she emphasized how little we know about the effects of Bt on the human diet. 'That research hasn't been done,' she said. I pressed. 'Is there any reason I shouldn't eat these spuds?' 'Let me turn that around. [she said,] Why would you want to?'" [17]

The uninvited houseguest

I wish I were done with the Bt story. Unfortunately, this product seems to infiltrate into a variety of issues, with inconclusive results. One of the issues is the ability of Bt to do exactly that: extend itself through the phenomenon of "genetic drift," a potentially serious problem. We should understand the science behind it before we look at its ramifications. Martin Teitel clearly explains why engineered pollen is so susceptible to "drift":

> When plants are genetically engineered to accept inserted, alien genes, those new genes are kept in a turned-on status. The inserted, engineered genes express their characteristics some or all of the time, instead of just once in a while. Further, the vectors, the biological airline that transports the inserted genes, are specially designed to move easily into new organisms — that, after all, is their purpose. So we end up with hyperactive genes carried by eager transport mechanisms. The result is a tendency of these genes to spread.
>
> Because the genes are designed to be on all the time, and because they have enthusiastic vectors for transport mechanisms, they can easily end up in neighboring crops, even organic ones. For some time the biotech industry has insisted that pollen cannot travel very far and so genetically modified characteristics would be confined to the fields of farmers who chose to use the technology. This assertion goes contrary to the experience of worried organic growers and farmers of non-genetically engineered crops, who by 1999 were starting to fail tests for GMO-free labels in Europe.[18]

Examples of gene pollution are popping up all over the place. Tom Wiley is one farmer who lost thousands of dollars in a deal with Japan due to the presence of uninvited GMOs. An article describes his experience: "Japan has a strict limit of one percent genetically modified beans in food grade products. Wiley thought this wouldn't be a problem, because he never had grown GM soybeans. However, test results came back showing that 1.37 percent of his beans were GM, so he lost that sale."[19]

Genetic drift is no longer just a business problem for conventional farmers, or even a certification problem for organic growers. This pollution has now wreaked havoc in an almost sacred gene pool area and has created the potential for an international conflict.

Michael Pollan writes, "Companies like Monsanto have long acknowledged that their engineered genes ('transgenes') might on rare occasions 'flow' by means of cross-pollination from one of their crops into neighboring plants. But because sex in nature takes place only between closely related species, and because most crop plants don't have close relatives in North America, the risk that new genetic traits would contaminate the genome of the world's important crops was, the companies claimed, remote. As long as genetically modified corn seed wasn't sold to Mexican farmers, or potato seed to Peruvians, these crucial 'centers of diversity' could be protected."[20]

> "Genetic drift is no longer just a business problem for conventional farmers, or even a certification problem for organic growers. This pollution has now wreaked havoc in an almost sacred gene pool area and has created the potential for an international conflict."

Guess where they have found GMOs? In Mexico! Planting GMO crops has been illegal in Mexico since 1998. An Associated Press article reported at the end of 2001 that samples revealed that just a few years of unlabeled US imports had transferred modified genes to local corn in the southern state of Oaxaca — even though planting genetically modified crops is banned in this country, the birthplace of corn. Mexicans, whose ancestors believed the gods created Man from an ear of corn, were outraged by the discovery.

A majority of the corn grown in the US comes from nine different varieties. This is minuscule compared with the 20,000 varieties and relatives of corn grown in Mexico. If more and more of these precious varieties are muffled out of existence by the GMO version, we lose much of the fallback source for classic corn-breeding for the future. We depend on these varieties in case of crop disaster or overwhelming pest invasions, so scientists may breed a variety that can withstand the enemy of the moment.

Many people have asked why environmentalists and other opponents of biotechnology become so very angry at the government and at the businesses that are simply trying to do what they do — develop products and sell them. One reason may be their almost exclusive focus on making money. When this potentially devastating mishap occurred in Mexico, Ricardo Celma, head of the Mexican office of the US Grain Council, made a statement (as reported in the Associated Press) that seemed more concerned with potential income loss for the biotech companies than for the potential devastation for Mexico. He said, "If a locally occurring variety receives some improvement from genetically engineered crops, it's up to the courts to decide whether farmers should be made to pay for that. But we want the patent rights of the owners of that genetic modification to be honored."

Mexico considers this pollution far from an improvement. "'The prospect of some multinational corporation bringing lawsuits against Mexican farmers would be intolerable,' the head of the Mexican government's Council on Biodiversity, Jorge Soberon, said Saturday." [21]

Bad behavior angers plenty

It is not just the Mexican authorities who are angered by such an insult. This type of news angers a lot of people. I gained a better understanding of biotechnology at about the same time as the Seattle WTO demonstrations. I concurred with many who watched from the sidelines and expressed frustration at the level of violence. Hadn't we, I thought at the time, learned about nonviolent action by now? Hadn't the message of peace been clearly established by Gandhi, Martin Luther King Jr., Thich Nhat Hanh, and others? What was happening here?

I will never condone violence. And yet, in the past few years, I have come to understand the level of rage the arrogance of some of the multinationals breeds in their adversaries. The idea that anyone could respond to leaders of a country whose symbol of spirituality may be destroyed in such a way is unacceptable to me. I feel embarrassed by the lack of respect. (Okay, I got that off my chest.)

One of my first real hands-on experiences with biotech came at the Northeast Sustainable Agriculture Working Group's Resource Harvest meeting in December 1998. The "Terminator technology" was a hot topic around the fringes of the meeting, and the group decided to craft a letter from the attendees of the conference (not the sponsoring organization) to petition against using public dollars to advance it. I learned that the Terminator technology simply stops the life of a plant after one season by terminating its ability to make seed. I saw how such a thing could make an otherwise calm person see red.

Brewster Kneen says, "The Terminator technology wants to play a dirty trick on the plant by violently manipulating (engineering) it so that its life drive is sterilized, or dead at puberty, so to speak. Thus the 'owner' of the seed gains total control of its 'intellectual property' by deciding when it will die, denying the life of the plant to anyone else, including the farmer who purchased and planted the seed." [22]

Farmers have traditionally saved seeds from one season to the next, especially on subsistence farms in poor, developing countries. As Vandana Shiva, an internationally known Indian scientist, environmentalist, and feminist, explained in a 1998 interview with *In Motion* magazine, "When we plant a seed there's a very simple prayer that every peasant in India says: 'Let the seed be exhaustless, let it never get exhausted, let it bring forth seed next year.' Farmers have such pride in saying 'this is the tenth generation seeds that I'm planting,' 'this is the fifth generation seed that I'm planting.' Just the other day I had a seed exchange fair in my valley and a farmer brought Basmati aromatic rice seed and he said 'this is five generations we've been planting this in our family'. So far human beings have treated it as their duty to save seed and ensure its continuity. But that prayer to let the seed be exhaustless seems to be changing into the prayer, 'let this seed get terminated so that I can make profits every year' which is the prayer that Monsanto is speaking through the Terminator technology — a technology whose aim is merely to prevent seed from germinating so that they don't have to spend on policing."[23]

An article in *New Scientist* described the inventor's reasoning for the product. "He [Melvin Oliver] claims that seeds manipulated in this way will grow into healthy plants that produce sterile seeds. He anticipates that it will be welcomed by seed companies, who regard the replanting of seeds as theft of their intellectual property. 'Our system is a way of self-policing the unauthorized use of American technology,' says Oliver. It's similar to copyright protection."[24]

And to think your tax dollars paid for part of this technology. The USDA and Delta Pine and Land were the partners on this innovation. Melvin Oliver, the inventor quoted above, was working at USDA labs! According to Oliver, "We provided 190,000 tax dollars (combined with Delta Pine's $530,000) to fund this revolutionary research."[25] Had the technology continued, the USDA would have earned royalties on the deal.

Knowing this, it is hard to read the following comments, also quoted in *New Scientist*, without serious skepticism: "Willard Phelps, a spokesman for the USDA, predicts that the new technique will soon be so widely adopted that farmers will only be able to buy seeds that cannot be regerminated. The US government's aim is merely to ensure the profits that are made from its introduction are not excessive, he says."[26]

Putting a patent on life

Monsanto raised the white flag on this particular battle at the end of 1999, when it announced it would make no effort to market the seeds that produce infertile crop plants, "for the foreseeable future." But they certainly did not stop the war. Another battle on the field is about GMO seeds being patented.

Actually, since a landmark Supreme Court ruling in the case of Diamond v. Chakrabarty in 1980, corporations have had the right to patent a range of organisms. Now farmers purchasing Monsanto seed must sign an agreement saying they will not use the seed except for the first growing season. They also pay a fee above and beyond the cost of the seed for technology transfer. Even though critics have argued non-stop, the ability to patent life through seed continues.

In a *Wall Street Journal* article in December 2001, Scott Kilman reported, "The US Supreme Court, in a ruling beneficial to the crop-biotechnology industry, upheld the patent-ability of plants and seed. The 6–2 opinion, which was closely watched by intellectual-property experts, keeps intact hundreds of utility patents granted by the US Patent and Trademark Office over the past 16 years to companies such as Monsanto Co. and DuPont Co.'s Pioneer Hi-Bred International Inc. unit."[27]

Ralph Nader shares his thoughts about the patenting of life: "Food — its economic, cultural, environmental, and political contexts — is one of the ultimate commonwealths. The ownership and control of the seeds of life, through exclusive proprietary technology shielded by corporate privileges and immunities, cannot be permitted in any democracy."[28] And some biotech critics think this behavior simply does not belong in our jurisdiction. One of those critics is Charles, the Prince of Wales, who said that the production of GM foods "takes mankind into realms that belong to God and to God alone."[29]

> "Food — its economic, cultural, environmental, and political contexts — is one of the ultimate commonwealths."

Vandana Shiva talks about the issue of "biopiracy." In essence the concept describes the multinationals' practice of taking plant material from cultures around the world, manipulating it, patenting it as "intellectual property," and selling it back to the culture from where it was taken in the first place ... for a fee. One story that extended my understanding of the damage done to these indigenous populations by "claiming" life comes from *Genetic Engineering: Changing the Nature of Nature*:

> Food-producing plants have never been the product of one person's work. The interaction between people and their food plants is subtle and long-range, sometimes taking hundreds of years or more to go from a tiny ear of corn the size of a finger to the foot-long sweet corn we buy in supermarkets, or from the grape-sized ancient tomatoes to the juicy behemoths that grace our summer gardens. A single variety of potato or wheat could be the result of a community's patient,

collective effort over scores of generations. It is the cooperative, communal nature of plant breeding that has made it part of the common heritage of humankind.

In more recent times, plant breeding has been taken on by big universities and corporations. These production-oriented entities have searched the globe for the raw material of their plant-breeding experiments, often using what they call "plant collection." In these "expeditions," botanists, agronomists, or anthropologists travel to distant countries, usually the nonindustrialized lands where the food plants originated. The collectors bring back samples to base their new varieties on. Although the plants that are "discovered" on these expeditions might be the result of thousands of years of patient community effort, the collectors just take and use. Why would they need to ask, they say, when after all the seeds or cuttings they bring home are the common heritage of humankind?

The problem arises when the universities, governments, or corporations that get the plants from other nations place strains of those plants, or processes using those plants, under patent. With the stroke of a pen (or, more likely, the press of a computer key), the common heritage of some distant people or tribe becomes the exclusive property of those who took it. Even the originators of the plant could risk infringement if they clashed with the patent holders in how they used their own foodstuffs — plants that had been passed down to them by their ancestors, plants that are intertwined with their cuisine, culture, and religion.

This is biopiracy, the expropriation of what should never be owned, and it is possible only through the patent system that establishes "intellectual property rights" over what was formerly no one's — or everyone's — property. As Vandana Shiva points out, 'Through intellectual property rights, an attempt is made to take away what belongs to nature, to farmers, and to women, and to term this invasion improvement and progress.'[30]

Brewster Kneen sums it up: "I think 'modern biotechnology' is a bad attitude — a bad attitude towards life, towards Creation, towards other cultures and other ways of knowing and experiencing the world."[31]

Golden rice – gift or GMO poster child?

For those very same cultures that have been under biopirate attack, the companies have a solution, one that will look very good in our eyes: yellow rice with genetically inserted vitamin A will solve a malnutrition problem for millions! I would like to believe this is exciting stuff. As a matter of fact, this very point halts my black-and-white thinking. I like this direction. I believe strongly that technology can be a source of solutions. Wouldn't it be wonderful if the life sciences companies really were focused on the most debilitating problems of our time? It would be, but alas there is "no market" for it. There is no financial stream to be ensured (on the short term.) Per Pinstrup-Andersen, director of the International Food Policy Research Institute (policy arm of the Consultive Group in International Agricultural Research), puts it flatly, "The private sector will not develop crops to solve poor people's problems, because there is not enough money in it."[32] If these brilliant minds refocused their attention, they might be able to think of more sound alternatives. That is just my overly-optimistic fantasy life kicking in.

You may be wondering, after *Time* magazine heralded the new rice on its Summer 2000 cover, what could possibly be wrong with saving a million kids a year? First, an enormous amount of foundation funding went into this discovery (I cannot help but think of the same amount working to the benefit of some of the grassroots organizations you will find in Chapter 20), and ultimately, it is "owned" through patents. The other thing that bothers me is something I heard a while ago from Vandana Shiva concerning Roundup-ready crops (bioengineered crops that are "immune" to that herbicide). In a BBC lecture series, she said, "When I was participating in the United Nations Biosafety Negotiations, Monsanto circulated literature to defend its herbicide-resistant Roundup-ready crops on grounds that they prevent 'weeds from stealing the sunshine.' But what Monsanto calls weeds are the fields of edible greens that provide vitamin A and prevent blindness in children and anemia in women."[33] Her point is that with one hand, they take it away and with the other, they sell it back. In another setting she said, "On the particular issue of vitamin-A rice, we have very simple alternatives to it. Just in the Indian state of Bengal, 150 greens which are rich in vitamin A are eaten and grown by the women."[34] Again, I understand and support solving problems with technology ... as long as the solution is actually viable. Michael Pollan pulls the lid off the dream technology with the following scenario:

"Consider this: an 11-year-old would have to eat 15 pounds of cooked golden rice a day — quite a bowlful — to satisfy his minimum daily requirements of vitamin A. Even if that were possible (or if scientists boosted beta-carotene levels), it probably wouldn't do a malnourished child much good, since the body can only convert beta-carotene into vitamin A when fat and protein are present in the diet. Fat and protein in the diet are, of course, precisely what a malnourished child lacks."[35]

Now you see the problem I have with saving a million kids a year with this product. Yellow rice just doesn't do it. The icing on this cake is the media heyday the biotech industry is having. A *New York Times* article on the subject shared the sentiments of Gordon Conway, president of the Rockefeller Foundation, which financed the original research on the golden rice: "'The public relations uses of golden rice have gone too far.' While genetically engineered rice has a role to play in combating malnutrition, Conway noted, 'We do not consider golden rice the solution to the vitamin-A deficiency problem.'"[36]

Remember, if you see those television commercials or print ads with adorable Asian children eating from a rice bowl, the message intimating that vitamin A rice will alleviate blindness and infection in millions of children, there are some caveats. According to a Washington Post article announcing the campaign in April 2000, "The biotechnology industry launched a preemptive strike yesterday, committing up to $50 million a year for a massive advertising campaign." The organization running the campaign is the Council for Biotechnology Information with funding from companies such as Monsanto, Aventis, Dow, and Dupont.[37]

Too late ... it's in our food

GMOs are in approximately 70 percent of our foods already. They got there, critics suggest, because the biotech companies focused on ingredients that are typically used in processed foods. They did not, after all, get a very good reception on their early whole vegetables — tomatoes or potatoes — so instead, they went to items we can't really see and don't think about very often. Soy and corn are grown for a variety of purposes. Besides the commonplace corn oil or soymilk, we don't think much about these ingredients. But "soy products appear in many processed and prepared foods. No one knows just how many of these products contain GMOs, but the words soybean oil, soy flour, isolated soy protein, textured vegetable protein, functional or nonfunctional soy protein concentrates, and textured soy protein concentrates on the label are good tipoffs." [38]

> ## Shopping tip
>
> *"No one knows just how many of these products contain GMOs, but the words soybean oil, soy flour, isolated soy protein, textured vegetable protein, functional or nonfunctional soy protein concentrates, and textured soy protein concentrates on the label are good tipoffs."*

Since the products are not labeled as "made with GMO ingredients," there is, of course, no way to tell which ones have it and which ones do not. To get a handle on it, states Teitel, "In 1997 the *New York Times* had Genetic ID of Fairfield, Iowa, test several foods to determine whether or not they contained genetically engineered ingredients. They tested four soy-based baby formulas and eight other products made with soy or corn. Most of the products contained hidden genfood."[39]

Several critics of biotech suggest this is a calculated plan on the part of the industry to intermingle our foods as quickly as possible before labeling takes affect. Then it will be too late and too expensive to try to segregate. When I first started to hear this argument, I wondered if the critics hadn't gone a bit overboard, until I read Brewster Kneen's personal encounter with the strategy:

In 1997 I participated in a seminar for high school teachers from across Canada, this one on the pros and cons of labeling GE foods. The North American PR official for AgrEvo, one of the big six agrotoxin/biotech companies, presented a detailed and absurd explanation to the teachers as to why it was impossible to segregate crops from GE seed and crops from conventional seed. Since segregation was impossible, she concluded, so was labeling. Then, to my amazement, she said, Besides which, once the horse is gone it is too late to fix the stable door! Being next on the panel, I could not help saying, Thank you very much Margaret [Gadsby]. I am glad that Ray [Mowling, Monsanto's vice-president] is also here, since you have just confirmed what I have long suspected, and if I am wrong you can tell me. What I have suspected is that you have an industry policy of getting as many GE crops through the regulatory process and on to the market — and into the supermarket — as fast as possible. I have also suspected that you have been pushing the deliberate mixing of GE and non-GE so that you can say, as you just did, it's too late to segregate and label. There was no comment.[40]

A *New York Times* article the summer of 2001 brought forth a near-admission of the strategy. As the story goes, "The United States, Brazil and Argentina account for about 90 percent of the world's corn and soybean exports. Bulk shipments from the United States and Argentina are predominately biotech. And Brazil is widely believed to have a black market in biotech soybeans. If Brazil legalizes biotech production, Europe and Asia — the world's two biggest purchasers of soy — would have almost nowhere to turn for adequate supplies of nonbiotech soybeans. 'We are very hopeful that last domino will fall,' said Bob Callanan, a spokesman for the

American Soybean Association, a trade group that supports the use of gene-altered crops."[41]

For a while there, it looked as if some farmers really didn't want to take the risk of losing overseas customers, and thus the amount of land dedicated to biotech crops might slowly erode. Unfortunately, figures from 2000 to 2001 show nothing but growth. The increase in global GM crop area grew 19 percent, almost twice the increase (11 percent) from the previous year (1999–2000). These aren't small numbers, either. According to the International Service for the Acquisition of Agri-Biotech Applications (ISAAA), the GM crop area in 2001 grew to 130 million acres. [42]

Looking for labels

No labeling. How can this possibly be? It certainly is not as if we don't care. A June 2001 ABC News poll indicated 93 percent of Americans want genetically engineered foods to be labeled. Nearly all respondents in the Rutgers University poll, 98 percent said foods created through GM processes should have special labels on them.

The government responded this past summer in a CBS News broadcast. "Labeling is very difficult," James Maryanski, head of biotech for FDA said. "Under the current law, we don't have authority that's broad enough to require labeling simply because consumers would like to have that information." Right now there may be no plans to require labeling.[43] What-ever! (I can see my daughter's up-turned-eyes and the slow sing-songy pronunciation, "What-ever." In today's youthful slang, it translates as, "You're nuts, but I am going along with it because I'm not going to get anywhere arguing with you because you are the authority.")

More essential to the argument against labeling is the government's declaration that the new versions are the same as the old versions. (By the way, I still don't understand how anything new is virtually old or unchanged, but, what-ever.) I guess not everyone in the government believes it: "In the US, private sector pressure led the White House to decree 'no substantial difference' between altered and normal seeds, thus evading normal FDA and EPA testing. Confidential documents made public in an on-going class action lawsuit have revealed that the FDA's own scientists do not agree with this determination."[44]

> "A June 2001 ABC News poll indicated 93 percent of Americans want genetically engineered foods to be labeled. Nearly all respondents in the Rutgers University poll, 98 percent said foods created through GM processes should have special labels on them."

As always, Michael Pollan seems to have a witty perspective: "In a dazzling feat of positioning, the industry has succeeded in depicting [GM] plants simultaneously as the linchpins of a biological revolution — part of a 'new agricultural paradigm' that will make farming more sustainable, feed the world and improve health and nutrition — and oddly enough, as the same old stuff, at least so far as those of us at the eating end of the food chain should be concerned."[45]

Various states have gotten into GMO labeling action, but none so far have agreed to mandatory labeling. The Pew Initiative on Food and Biotechnology reported, "In fact, in 2001, 36 states considered some kind of legislation related to genetically modified (GM) food and agricultural biotechnology... At present, no states require a level of review and approval more rigorous than federal regulations. In 2001, however, a few states (Maine, Maryland, and North Dakota) passed bills that attempt to place stronger and more specific controls on the use of GM crops."[46] More information on state biotech legislative status is available on the website **<http://pewagbiotech.org/>**.

I hope the labeling laws will have changed considerably by the time you read this book. The US trails other countries on labeling. Although the US clearly argues for biotech in many international trade disputes, it seems that globalization will probably demand some level of consistency on this issue. At this point, as reported in the *Vancouver Sun*, "The European Union, Japan, South Korea, Australia, and Mexico require mandatory labeling of GM foods .... Canada is a little ahead of the US — Canada is getting close to acceptance. In October [2001], a required mandatory labeling bill was defeated 126 to 91 in Canada."[47]

The most recent disappointment in the US labeling effort is the FDA's crackdown on non-GMO language. The industry is concerned that people will assume a non-GMO product is superior. After reading this chapter, you might be nodding your head. From an article in the *Wall Street Journal*: "'We want to stop misleading statements,' said Christine Taylor, director of the FDA office that supervises label claims. It's far from clear, however, exactly what a food company can legally say about its efforts to avoid biotechnology. The agency is still wading through 55,000 public comments on the wording guidance it wants to issue to companies."[48]

While they wade, let's finish up with a quick look at some of the campaigns being waged by various groups.

Join the effort!

To stay on top of this urgent issue, check out the many organizations out there doing good work. This handful of groups and their websites is intended to give you a starting point for your foray into biotechnology.

- **The Campaign to Label Genetically Engineered Foods** is out of Seattle, Washington. They have an excellent "Take Action Packet" that can be purchased in bulk for sharing with friends who "need to know." **<www.thecampaign.org>**

- **The Center for Food Safety** in Washington, DC, has a tremendous amount of information available on its website and is a good place to get your voice heard. **<www.foodsafetynow.org>**

- **Greenpeace** in Washington, DC, has a fantastic list of name brand items on "The Greenpeace True Food Shopping List," which fall into two categories: green for go-ahead, or red for no-go — GMOs. **<www.truefoodnow.org>**

- **Mothers for Natural Law** is based in Fairfield, Iowa and maintains a list of non-GE products and primary suspects on their "What to Eat and How to Shop" link. **<www.safe-food.org>**

- **The Turning Point** project in Washington, DC, is responsible for those public service print ads against GMOs (and other things), and it also gives a partial list of biotech foods. **<www.turnpoint.org>**

11

All Creatures Great and Small

YESTERDAY I SPOKE WITH OUR LAND GRANT EXTENSION LIVESTOCK ADVISOR about some of my concerns. He assured me that some of the stories I am about to share are overreactions. He pulled out charts and pictures and even genetic code language to try to help me see the truth. We are on different sides of many environmental discussions. In the end, we did, however, agree on one overriding concept. The science is not evil by itself; it is the questionable ethical application of that science that causes problems.

A great example is the announcement in August 2001 that University of Guelph scientists had figured out how to develop a genetically engineered pig that would excrete less phosphorus, reducing the effects of pig manure on the environment. Quickly patented (oh, yes, animals and human genes may receive patents, too, once they have been genetically engineered) as "Enviropigs," the sow gives pork producers a public relations tool to counter concerns about the serious contamination caused by confinement farming.

Clare Schlegal, chairman of Ontario Pork, a trade association representing 4,400 pig farmers in that Canadian province, said, "Pork producers are being looked at as polluters — this is one technology to show that we do care."[1] Instead of facing the real issue, too many pigs in too small a space, they have sought a technological advancement to protect the current practices. There are other ways to reduce phosphorous levels, but they are interdisciplinary (from different disciplines) and don't work like a silver bullet. They would take consistent stewardship.

There are stewards, but before we get to them, let's look a little more deeply at what's happening down on the farm. Genetic engineering of livestock is not on the front burner at the moment. On-farm stewardship is. So, what is happening down on the farm? First of all, you would hardly consider calling it a farm anymore. These are not scenes from *Charlotte's Web* or the movie *Babe*. These are huge agribusinesses that squeeze too many animals into too little space.

Raise the roost!

The livestock advisor showed me photographs of one of the homes of broiler chickens (the ones we eat versus the layers that give us eggs). In the first picture, they appeared to be in early adolescence, not really chicks, but not big white fluffy birds yet either, and they seemed to have quite a bit of room. Chickens like to flock, so they were all together in one area, but it clearly looked as if they could roam freely around the open space, the size of a football field. The photo showing the full-grown version gave a clear picture of overcrowding. I couldn't tell if the birds could spread their wings, but it certainly did not look comfortable. It also didn't seem to provide them with the opportunity to peck the ground, a behavior experts say is important to chickens. According to the Humane Society of the US, "20,000 to 30,000 'broiler' chickens are crowded together inside one building up to 400 feet long; individual buildings house more than 100,000 egg-laying hens, and keeping one to two million birds on a single site is becoming increasingly common."[2] That is an awful lot of chickens. As I think how often my family has chicken, from pasta dishes and whole chickens to chicken salads, it is not all that surprising. As North Americans have reduced consumption of red meats of all kinds, chicken has taken over as a virtual staple in our lives.

Then consider the amount of chicken used at restaurants, particularly fast-food restaurants with nuggets and sandwiches, then add in the hens kept to produce eggs, and the numbers shortly become astronomical. John Robbins, in his new book, *The Food Revolution*, describes the animal welfare issues McDonald's has faced over the past five or so years. After battling activists and technically winning but receiving bad publicity in what is now referred to as the McLibel trial in Great Britain, McDonald's was further challenged by People for the Ethical Treatment of Animals (PETA). Following that multi-year combat, McDonald's adopted slightly improved conditions for the chickens that supplied them with eggs. "The new guidelines called for chickens to have more space then they did previously (from an average of seven to eight hens per 18-inch-by-20 inch cage to a maximum of five), and for the elimination of 'forced molting' (the starving of hens in order to increase egg production). At the same time, McDonald's called for chickens to be caught more humanely prior to slaughter, and they started auditing slaughterhouses. And for the first time in its history, McDonald's threatened to cut off suppliers who were not in compliance with humane slaughter guidelines."[3]

I hear mixed reactions to this news. Some say McDonald's was forced into the new behavior and not to give them too much credit. Others say it was a real success, the first step in modeling improved conditions. And finally, some express frustration at how little improvement it really is. In *Orion* magazine, last winter, the reality of the changes was made clear. "However praiseworthy, these new measures fail to address fundamental questions regarding our relation to the animals we raise."[4] The new guidelines expanded the area provided per bird layers' cages from the size of a Kleenex box to that of a brownie pan.[5]

To be truthful, I can't bear to share many of the stories of the confinement and brutality of livestock raising. Does this mean every factory farmer is cruel? Of course not. My argument is not with the individual farmer, but with the standard practices that tend to squeeze every penny out of production. Farmers are under contract with large corporations. The Humane Society of the US (HSUS) reports, "Virtually all poultry raised in the US are under contract … studies show that the large poultry companies reap a 20–30 percent return on their investment. The most contract growers can hope for is a 1–3 percent return despite the fact that the growers invest more than 50 percent of the entire capital in the industry. Studies also show that more than 80 percent of poultry farmers' earnings are below poverty level."[6] Forget the image of the old fashioned farmer with a straw hat and overalls spending quality time with his chickens. With statistics like these, I am sure you can conjure up your own unfortunate picture.

Huge corporations produce 98 percent of all poultry in the US.[7] What happened to our chicken farmers? You have heard about many of them in news reports about the disappearance of family farms. Writer Melanie Adcock of the HSUS described the situation in 1993. "In the past twelve years, 80 percent of US egg producers have been driven out of business. This loss of farmers has paralleled the increase in the number of producers keeping more than a million birds, all in battery cages."[8]

How does all this relate to our purchases? Let's begin with eggs. I look for free-range or locally grown (if you know the farmer is not using factory-type practices).

Organic in this case means the chickens have been fed organic grain, so you cannot be assured they have had an opportunity to walk around (although it may be more likely). About 98 percent of supermarket eggs are produced by hens that live up to two years crowded into tiny cages with other hens.[9] If you can't find free-range eggs, ask your grocer to stock them. Along with eggs, you might also look for free-range chicken broth. A number of new products offer hens a better life. Can I guarantee that the companies saying they offer a free-range opportunity actually do? No, but it will send a message, anyway.

What about the chicken we eat? There are two major issues here; the first pertains to animal welfare. We want natural chickens that have had a chance to live a normal life. While in the past, a broiler reached its 4-pound market weight in 21 weeks, today's birds, deliberately bred for obesity [or excessive muscle growth], take only seven weeks to reach the same weight.[10] The problems associated with these "super chickens" are endless. According to Michael Appleby of the Humane Society, "Slow-growing birds with more exercise produce meat with better taste and texture."[11] Unfortunately, at this point, there really is no labeling that lets us know we have a slow-growing or traditional chicken. Your best bet is to find a local farmer with more space and less pressure to follow factory farming practices. Plenty of farms just outside urban areas sell to independent grocers inside the city limits. Try to seek them out.

> ## Shopping tip
>
> *"Unfortunately, at this point, there really is no labeling that lets us know we have a slow-growing or traditional chicken. Your best bet is to find a local farmer with more space and less pressure to follow factory farming practices."*

The second issue is the use of antibiotics, discussed in Chapter 2. Antibiotic use is not limited to the poultry business; it is also happening with pigs and cattle. As reported by the Institute of Agriculture and Trade Policy, "The majority of these animals are routinely given subtherapeutic doses of antibiotics to make them grow faster and convert feed to flesh more efficiently. Low-level antibiotic feed additives are also used to control disease in animals that are raised under less than optimal environmental and management conditions."[12]

The other night, I noticed a discarded *Time* magazine on my husband's side of the bed. We fight over it — I lost this week. It was an updated health issue with a story entitled, "Playing Chicken With Our Antibiotics: overtreatment is creating dangerously resistant germs."[13] My first reaction was, Great! The story is in mainstream press — maybe we will have more antibiotic-free chicken in the future. My second reaction was, What a nifty title! It really says it all. We are taking too much risk and will ultimately lose. As the article says, "Chicken Cipro [remember from Chapter 2, we have been giving poultry the anthrax cure] is only the latest example of how humans are burning their pharmacological bridges. Feedlot operators are dosing their livestock with antibiotics to keep them healthy under stressful conditions."[14]

The details go like this: the chicken Cipro is a drug called Enroflaxin, in a class of antibiotics called fluoroquinolones. From a press release by the group Environmental Defense: "Physicians have used fluoroquinolones as an essential treatment for foodborne disease (particularly on campylobacter bacteria) since 1986. Very little resistance occurred until its use in poultry began in 1995. By 1998, the Centers for Disease Control found that over 13 percent of foodborne campylobacter was resistant to fluoroquinolones. Last year resistance rose to nearly 18 percent."[15]

Why are chicken farmers using antibiotics? For a myriad of reasons, many related to the overcrowding of factory farms. Suffice it to say, demand antibiotic-free chicken at your local grocer and read on for more about why antibiotics are so often used in factory farming.

> ### Shopping tip
> *"Suffice it to say, demand antibiotic free chicken at your local grocer and read on for more about why antibiotics are so often used in factory farming.*

A load of hogwash

Nearly 93 percent of pigs in the United States receive antibiotics in the diet at some time during the grow/finish period.[16] One reason for subtherapeutic use (less than the amount given when treating an all out illness) is stress. Think about how much easier it is to come down with a cold or flu when you are stressed out. Farmers want to avoid taking a sick animal out of operation, but there is a risk that the illness will spread to all the animals. They hedge their bets with antibiotics.

The National Research Council found that the prophylactic effect of subtherapeutic antibiotics is less pronounced in clean, healthful, stress-free environments, while their beneficial effects are greatest in poor sanitary conditions.[17] You would be stressed, too, if you were raised on metal slats with hardly enough room to turn around. Why the metal slats? When the animal urinates and defecates, (most of) the waste falls between the slats into a man-made river, transporting it to huge manure lagoons.

My husband and I raised a pair of pigs a couple of years ago. I noticed they were somewhat fastidious. I don't think they would be very happy standing in their own excrement. They love to root around, and their sense of smell is highly sensitive. In France, pigs are used to sniff out truffles underground, so I can only imagine they must be miserable when raised under such conditions.

Slaughter

The slaughterhouse sits on top of the highest hill around. Both entrances, people's and animals', face the view across a meadow rich with fall colors: green and gold grasses broken occasionally by fallen, weathered tree trunks and studded here and there with brown boulders. A white cow grazes, and beyond her the meadow tumbles down into an iridescent valley of foliage. It is a day to be grateful just for being alive.

The two pigs I have brought to slaughter are in the back of the pickup, lying on a bed of straw under a camper top. They have no names, because everyone agreed naming them would strengthen any attachment we might develop with them. They have made the 45-minute trip with little fussing.

Last spring, raising pigs seemed a nearly perfect idea. They would eat the poison ivy that prevented us from cultivating a patch of ground. They would eat our leftovers and spoiled food, becoming the ultimate composters. We would have meat without contributing to the worldwide crisis of grain-to-meat nutrition loss. We would join the historical circle of farmers who've raised a yearly pig, among them the eminently sensible E.B. White. We would enhance our self-sufficiency.

But most of all, I said, we would force ourselves into awareness of the real relationship we've always had, but never felt, with the animals we have eaten. Never before had I looked in the eye of the animals I consumed. I joked, about getting the pigs, "We'll either eat them or we'll become vegetarians."

I go inside to make my arrangements. I'm in a small butcher shop next to a cooler full of steaks and hot dogs and other cuts, and a few local cheeses.

At the end is a small counter and a cash register. For a moment I'm buoyed by the evidence of smallness of scale. The animals that gave this meat were fed by people, not machines. They were no doubt kept in pens large enough to move in. Their meat will be eaten by the same people who raised them, implying a level of awareness inaccessible to customers in a supermarket.

I place my order with a woman in a bloodstained butcher's apron: cut the hams in half, cut the pork chops an inch thick, slice the bacon, save the fatback for soap. I pay my $120, and the woman tells me to take the pigs around to the holding pen.

When the pigs arrived in June, none of us were prepared for dealing with personalities. The first proof that these were sentient beings was their fear. They cowered against the back of the little moveable pen I'd built as a temporary home for them. They were small, no more than two feet long, a female and a male. The male had been castrated, said Dan, which shocked me. No one had told me this would happen, but why would they? I hadn't known even what gender the pigs would be or how old. All I knew was that I'd given Dan a check for $90 for two pigs.

After fear, the piglets revealed their determination. They spent nearly every waking minute digging up the ground of their pen with their snouts. It took them just one day to turn their four-by-eight patch of lawn into cratered dirt. Day by day I moved their pen up the fence line; they ate our poison ivy and ruined their strip of lawn.

I encountered their drive for freedom one morning on my way to feed them before work. They were gone. I thought they'd buried themselves under the straw as they had before, but they hadn't – they just weren't there. Then I heard a snort on the other side of the fence. The piglets sauntered sleepily from under the tall grass and skunk cabbage, where they'd apparently spent the night, and walked through the gate I held open for them. Now that they had the run of the enclosed lawn, they made the most of it. Cyn and I, dressed in our fancy work suits, and she in heels, chased them around the lawn for a few minutes while the kids whooped it up on the deck, watching for us to be outmaneuvered. This was fun for the piglets, too. Like children, they kept it up until the adults' refusal to play got boring, then they moped into the pen.

They got out often after that, even after we moved them to the big pen on the other side of the lawn fence, even after they were huge, no matter how many extra stakes I drove to secure the hog fencing. One day they stopped traffic on the road in front of our house.

The holding pen is a concrete room at the other end of the building. Several animals wait there already, separated into a few enclosures by tubular livestock gates tied together at the corners. The animals make no sound. They are still. I can feel their disorientation. A man comes through the holding pen from the slaughterhouse to help me. He wears high rubber boots. I imagine he's the one who will kill them.

I've been told this place might mistreat animals, and I have agonized over this for days. I'm anxious to make contact with this man, to evoke kindness for my pigs. "How's it going?" I ask. He looks at me, a little surprised and a little open. "I've had better days," he says, clearly wanting to say more. This is a man in deep depression. "It's just ... " he falters and shrugs, " ... it's just life, I guess." I'm surprised he's sharing his pain so openly – a good sign, I guess, and I try to commiserate, "It's tougher than ever to make it these days." I wonder if he is depressed because he makes his living killing his fellow creatures.

When the piglets had been with us for only a couple of days, they began to greet us whenever we appeared. They barked and jumped around their pen like puppies. When Cynthia and the children returned home each noontime and walked onto the back deck, the pigs heard the sliding door open and gave them the same reception. In October, when the pigs weighed more than 150 pounds each and seemed too big to run, they still careened around the pen in greeting. The person they knew best was our next-door neighbor. She visited them often, and they loved to touch noses with her dogs through the fence. She showed me one day how she could scratch one of them behind the ear until he swooned and plopped his rump to the ground, holding his head up for more. "I'm so sorry they have to go," she said.

In their last few days, I kept trying to achieve the relationship with them I'd hoped for all along. I wanted to emulate the native peoples I'd heard about, to thank the pigs for feeding me and my family, to show them respect and understand our roles as life-giver and blessed life-sharer. I wanted communion. But it didn't happen. I felt only separation, guilt, and dread. "They're giving up their lives," I said to Cynthia one night as we went to bed.

Don and I open the tailgate to unload the pigs. They cower against the front of the truck bed. I grab one of their front legs and pull. He wrenches away. I grab an ear. Desperate to get it over with, I pull hard, and then I'm shocked that I'm willing to hurt him in this of all moments, so I let go of his ear. I grab both front legs. He moves close enough for me to wrap my arms around his neck in a kind of embrace. I pull him the rest of the way to the tailgate and ease him onto the loading dock. The second pig follows, with only a little coaxing.

The man opens the stock gate a bit, and the first pig walks calmly toward the opening. I hear an animal scream briefly inside the building. The man takes an oversized stick of orange chalk and scrawls my initials on the back of the first pig. Reading from behind the animal, I watch him draw a large fluorescent "L" just behind the shoulders and then a "B" just below it toward the rump. I feel like he's making an entry in the Book of Life. The pig makes his way into the pen and touches noses through a stock gate with the other pigs in there. The man scrawls "LB" on the second pig, and suddenly both pigs are inside. There's no time to say goodbye – a foolish thought, anyway, I tell myself. I hadn't been able to connect with them before; how could I possibly now? And this is no place to grieve – my business is done here. It's time to go.

Cynthia joined me on the trip to the slaughterhouse a week later to pick up the frozen meat. She wouldn't get out of the car, the place frightened her so. We rode home without a word about the pigs.

It has been three weeks since I delivered the pigs, and I'm still sickened at the thought of eating meat – Cynthia, too, though we've both had chicken a couple of times. The pork is still in our freezer, but we've made arrangements to sell it on consignment through Brookfield Farm, the community-supported farm we belong to.

The other day I needed to work through lunch, and I asked a co-worker to bring me a sandwich from the restaurant she was going to. After she left, I realized I had reflexively asked her for ham and cheese. By the time she returned, I was famished and I ate it. It made me nauseous.

Lee Barstow, November 1997

Industry statistics sadden me. Each year more than $87 million is lost because of poor meat quality, a direct result of stress, fatigue, and injuries; and at least 20 percent of factory-farmed pigs die in the intensive husbandry systems. [18] Stories of brutality are beyond my ability to share.

> **"At least 20 percent of factory-farmed pigs die in the intensive husbandry systems. Stories of brutality are beyond my ability to share."**

In 2001, Robert F. Kennedy, Jr. (whose message has been primarily environmental, but has recently expanded to include animal welfare) spearheaded an effort to force one of the big hog corporations to face its legal duty to clean up its act. In a public gathering initiating the campaign, Kennedy expressed his view of the matter. "'The way that we treat animals — somebody at sometime is going to be punished for that — we as a nation or somebody. Because you can't treat another work of the Creator with the kind of indignity that we are allowing to go on in this state or others without there being some kinds of karmic retribution at some point in history. I think all of us understand that, and particularly the family farmers here who understand the notion of stewardship and how an animal should be treated with dignity if we want dignity for ourselves.'"[19]

Remember, this way of farming is not being devised by farmers. As in the poultry industry, contract farming is taking hold. Economists estimate 50 percent of hogs slaughtered in 1999 were produced or sold under some form of contract.

"Between 1950 and 1999, the number of US farms selling hogs declined from 2.1 million to 98,460. In 1950, average sales per farm were around 31 hogs. By 1999, average sales had grown to around 1,100 market hogs per farm. One hundred and five farms having over 50,000 pigs each accounted for 40 percent of the US hog inventory.[20]

"The 1998 annual pig crop was 105,004,000, a record high."[21] And yet, the farmers don't earn a respectable living. The following story from an Institute for Agriculture and Trade Policy report, "The Price We Pay for Corporate Hogs" about who made the money in 1998, is replayed throughout industrial agriculture. "The record high hog supplies of 1998 [105,004,000] had hit a wall. Retailers did not lower prices to consumers; meatpackers and processors reduced their prices to farmers; specialized and highly capitalized hog factories could not easily reduce supply. The results were high marketing margins and record profits for the packing industry. While independent farmers were receiving the lowest prices since the Great Depression, Smithfield Foods, IBP, and Hormel Foods (first, second, and fifth largest hog packers, respectively) announced record profits."[22]

A whole lot more hogwash

Giant livestock farms, or "factory farms," housing hundreds of thousands of pigs, chickens, or cows, create huge amounts of waste, more than 130 times the amount that people do — about 2.7 trillion pounds of manure a year.[23] One hog factory in Missouri produces as much fecal waste as would a city of 360,000 people. The sheer amount of excrement is in and of itself a huge problem. Add to that stressful factory farming methods, and another problem is created: stressed animals pass more pathogens into their feces than do unstressed animals, and these pathogenic bacteria are the antibiotic-resistant ones.[24]

In addition, more than 40 diseases can be transferred to humans through animal manure.[25] How bad can it be? The farmer must simply store the manure somewhere, properly compost it (killing off the lion's share of the pathogens), and send it (in small quantities mixed with organic inputs) back to the fields. Right? Wrong. First, let's look at where farmers are "simply storing" it.

The most common solution is what are known as "manure lagoons." These lagoons emit serious air pollution into their local communities. Asthma and other serious illnesses abound in these towns. For "environmental" reasons, the lagoons are kept contained within clay structures to avoid harm to the groundwater. The lagoons are periodically drained and transferred to surrounding fields, not composted and without any balancing ingredients, moving the health hazards toward the foods we eat.

The normal everyday maintenance of these lagoons is not environmentally friendly. The emptying and refilling of the lagoons degrades their sidewalls over time, and eventually their clay liners can no longer prevent seepage. The worst damage occurs during flooding.

North Carolina, the number one state for hog production in the US, has had its share of floods. You may remember the media hoopla after Hurricane Floyd hit that state in 1999, when at least five manure lagoons burst and 47 were completely flooded.[26] That particular storm followed a long list of others.

"In June 1995, 25 million gallons of liquid manure broke through the berm surrounding a hog lagoon in Onslow County, North Carolina. The manure flowed over a neighbor's cropland and into the New River, creating the biggest lagoon spill on record and eventually killing 10,000,000 fish. The spill caused the closing of 364,000 acres of coastal wetland to shell fishing. The day before, a million-gallon hog lagoon spill had occurred in Sampson County. Later that same year, four more spills occurred in North Carolina, including 8.6 million gallons of liquid manure that spilled from poultry farms. In July 1996, floodwater from Hurricane Bertha led to a 1.8 million gallon spill from a hog waste lagoon in Craven County, North Carolina. In September 1996, Hurricane Fran caused the Cape Fear River to rise, flooding sewage treatment plants and manure lagoons and resulting in $6 billion in damages, $872 million of which were in farm losses. However, the worst was still to come. In September 1999, Hurricane Dennis hit North Carolina with eight inches of pounding rains, raising the levels of wastewater in hog lagoons. A week later, early on the morning of September 16, Hurricane Floyd brought 22 inches of rain. Floyd caused widespread flooding; drowned hogs, chickens, and turkeys; covered hog manure lagoons throughout Eastern North Carolina; and spread hog waste, rotting animal carcasses, and pathogens in the floodwaters."[27]

That was probably more than you wanted to hear. But isn't our biggest problem the fact that we don't want to hear it? We don't want pig farms to come to our towns — they wreak havoc on communities — but we want our bacon for breakfast, our ham for lunch, our pork chops for supper, and our pork tenderloin and crown roasts for special occasions. As the *New York Times* put it, "Defenders of the big hog plants, where thousands of hogs are confined in small pens, say the producers can scarcely be blamed for delivering the kind of lean, low-cost pork that American consumers demand."[28]

> **"I am not trying to shame anyone into being a vegetarian. I am not a vegetarian today. I have been before, and I probably will be again. I *am* trying to say we need to become more aware of these issues in our daily food choices."**

I am not trying to shame anyone into being a vegetarian. I am not a vegetarian today. I have been before, and I probably will be again. I *am* trying to say we need to become more aware of these issues in our daily food choices. Going further, we can also influence legislation and inform rural communities that are considering the lure of lucrative hog production. We could share the lessons learned in North Carolina. After the pounding that state went through, it has finally put its foot down to increased production facilities and further environmental contamination. Meanwhile, the hog industry is finding new locations where land is cheap and rules are few: states such as Idaho and Utah, countries such as Canada and Poland, and even Native American reservations.[29] Unfortunately, North Carolina must face the legacy of hog farms, with more than 700 abandoned manure lagoons festering like sores on its landscape.[30]

I recently heard a story about what might be a milestone for small hog farmers. On the way to tour an Amish farm, Glenda Yoder of Farm Aid (a wonderful organization known to consumers for its support of family farms, its annual Willie Nelson, Neil Young, and John Mellancamp and others concert/fundraisers, and known to sustainable agriculture groups as a great donor), told me about an enormous effort they had been supporting. It was about the Campaign for Family Farms, a group of pig farmers who were fed up with the federally mandated pork check-off fees. For every $100 of hog revenue, a farmer has to pay 45¢ to the National Pork Board. Most of these funds go to the National Pork Producers Council, which supports research and consumer marketing for the pork industry — but most of this supports the efforts of the big factory farms, not the little guys.

So a group of pig farmers who were fed up with these federally mandated pork check-off fees formed the Campaign for Family Farms. They rose up together and said, "No!" After bringing the USDA thousands of names on a petition calling for a referendum, a vote was conducted and passed, 53 percent to 47 percent, to make the check-off voluntary.

But the celebrations were cut short with the entry of the Bush administration. The *New York Times* reported the temporary end to this story with the article, "Unpopular Fee Makes Activists of Hog Farmers" in June 2001: "Ms. Ann M. Veneman, US Agriculture Secretary, said in an interview that she saw the vote differently. She said she threw it out because her lawyers said it was "procedurally flawed" and would not stand up to a court challenge filed by National Pork Producers Council officials the day after they lost the vote. The Council won a temporary restraining order against repealing the fee. But instead of carrying on the fight, she approved a settlement with the Council, promising to conduct a new survey of farmers in 2003 and to change procedures for spending the money."[31] Needless to say, after a three-year-plus fight, the farmers almost won. In the midst of all the hog industry's mess, I certainly want to join efforts with these farmers in 2003 to resist factory farms.

What about a Mad burger?

To all vegetarians reading this, please excuse me for a moment. I have always loved a good, juicy burger cooked at home on the grill, served with corn on the cob, a fresh salad of mixed greens, and a fresh baguette. Lately I have found those occasions to be far less frequent.

The meat industry has tried to turn cows into carnivores. With nowhere else to turn after detergents appeared on the scene, rendering houses gave up the soap business and turned to making feed out of animals — parts of animals, sick animals, animals that died for unknown reasons. This ended up being a handy way to increase the protein level of an animal's diet.

This practice is thought to have contributed to the contagious nature of Mad Cow disease. Remember a few years ago when all you saw on the television news were clips of burning carcasses in Britain? The disease is formally known as bovine spongiform encephalopathies (BSE). It basically eats away at its victim's brain, creating holes that ultimately look like a sponge. It has a long incubation period, from 10 to 30 years, after which it brings about dementia and finally death.

The research into this disease is still not complete, and some scientists think it is connected with an unorthodox protein — a prion. But clearly, feeding infected parts of one animal to many other animals is not terribly smart when the infection is widely contagious. Britain banned this practice in 1988, but the US was much slower to act.

The first case of the disease was found in Britain in 1985. For ten years, British authorities defended the safety of the meat supply, until it appeared the disease might be spreading to humans. According to Claude Fischler, it was "March 20, 1996 when the British government solemnly announced in the House of Commons that scientists closely following the epidemiology of Creutzfeldt-Jakob Disease [the human version of Mad Cow] had identified 10 cases [later to become 12] of what seemed to be a new form of the illness … according to the scientists, the most likely cause for this variant of CJD was contamination by the BSE agent before 1989."[32]

Creutzfeldt-Jacob Disease (nvCJD) results in a horrible death. As of 2002, more than 100 British victims and at least one in France have died from the human version of the disease. New studies suggest that a percentage of Alzheimer's victims have actually had nvCJD. This is a little too much for me to bear; I have a close friend with Alzheimer's disease. But before I consider this connection any further, I will look for more research beyond the two small studies conducted to date.

Another study released by the US Agriculture Department in 2001 and reported in the *New York Times* in November 2001, found little risk of Mad Cow disease being contracted by American cattle or of its ever posing a public health problem for humans.[33] This might be very good news, but media coverage said that scientists were questioning the study's results and that the Harvard Center, where the research was conducted, had received money from the industries under study.

With the enormity of the problem, I am sure new information will be available by the time you read this book. It might be best to keep up to date.

Got milk?

Dairy cows are often put through the same grueling life as beef cattle. While a dairy cow's natural lifespan is 20 to 25 years, animals raised under modern conditions are lucky to live four years. In a natural situation, a cow produces enough milk to feed one or two calves, but today's factory cows actually produce 20 times that amount.[34] Such "milk machines" produce an average of 15,567 pounds of milk a year, almost 40 percent more than a dairy cow would have produced just 16 years ago.[35] How does she do this? A variety of methods have been used to increase production of milk, one of which is to inject genetically produced growth hormone.

Synthetic recombinant bovine growth hormone (rBGH), also known as bovine somatotropin (BST) and trademarked by Monsanto as Posilac, is injected into milk cows every two weeks to boost milk production. However, it also increases the incidence of mastitis, an infection of the udder, which can contribute pus to milk. Pus in milk can reduce, or destroy, the commercial value of the milk, so farmers fight mastitis by treating their cows with antibiotics. In addition to mastitis, rBGH causes a short life span, and it leads to an increase in IGF-1, a hormone associated with an increased likelihood of cancer (breast, colon, and prostate) in humans. This hormone is not eliminated during pasteurization, so it may be passed on to the consumer.

> "A variety of methods have been used to increase production of milk, one of which is to inject genetically produced growth hormone."

One leader of the battle against rBGH is Samuel S. Epstein, M.D., whose book *Got (Genetically Engineered) Milk?: The Monsanto rBGH/BST Milk Wars Handbook* describes all the political ins and outs of the conflict over this hormone and the story behind the Fox Network debacle. Two television journalists tried to tell the story about the growth hormone on the Fox network, but pressure from the manufacturers shut them down. The story was watered down, and litigation has been filed. What appeared to be successful litigation against the network by the two "whistleblowers" has resulted in years of appeals.

Many countries have banned the use of rBGH, including Canada. According to a Consumers Union press release, the product is legal in the US, Mexico, and South Africa. The US has tried to

Shopping tip

"So unless you are a Canadian milk drinker, you might want to seek out an rBGH/BST-free label. If you prefer a local dairy, ask if it uses rBGH, and if it says yes … say no, thank you."

persuade international trade bodies to allow its use, but Codex Alimentarius (the UN's main food safety group) has so far blocked the attempts.

So unless you are a Canadian milk drinker, you might want to seek out an rBGH/BST-free label. If you prefer a local dairy, ask if it uses rBGH, and if it says yes … say no, thank you.

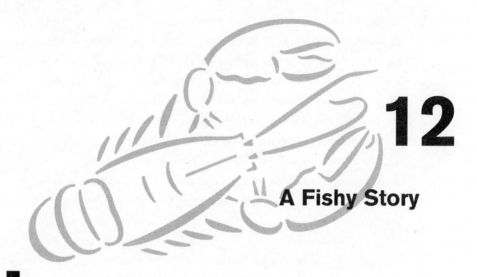

12

A Fishy Story

IT'S A ROMANTIC IMAGE, ONE THAT CAN STILL BE SEEN SOMETIMES: the solitary fisherman heading out to sea for the day in the early morning hours in a small fishing boat. Today's reality extends a few thousand miles offshore, where $40 million supertrawlers the size of a football field spend months searching with global positioning systems, clearing the deep waters and ocean floors with huge nets. Their catch is everything from tiny "junk" fish to an occasional endangered seal to the dinner on our plates, 400 tons of fish in a single netting.[1]

Sound familiar? The small, sustainable, local fishermen are just like farmers, losing out to huge fisheries with multimillion investments (some of which were paid for, in part, by our tax dollars) in excessive equipment and technology. According to a story in *Orion* in 2001, "Since 1995, nearly 80 New England fishing families, many from Gloucester, have sold their boats to the government as part of a $25 million federal buyout."[2]

Our wilds wear out

As with the farming industry, a few big companies control ever more products and elements of production. In the case of fishing, however, there is not another season to plant. When the companies exhaust the ocean of her fish, that's it. Between

A lobster shell

During my elementary school summers, I took late-afternoon adventures by myself down to the "pound." The lobster pound in South Bristol, Maine, was owned by one of the old fishing families in town. Every August, after a day at Christmas Cove, my mom and I would drive down the hill to the pound to select that night's lobsters. My friends generally weren't served lobster; either they didn't like it, or it was considered too much for children. I was lucky to always get my own … one of few advantages of being an only child.

These solitary adventures were more than an education – they expressed a culture I knew, even then, was rare and not to last for much longer. The men would arrive with the day's catch and empty their boats of mounds of fresh lobster, along with a few things that had ended up coming along for the ride. (I have since learned that those things, small, undesirable fish or sea animals, plus more unusual items, are considered "bycatch.") I would sit on the out-of-the-way traps watching keenly, but sure to stay out of the way.

I could tell it was a hard life, but the neighborhood lobstermen were nothing but kind – sometimes a little gruff, but always kind. I would ask a million questions, and they would share their stories.

There was a difference between the summer people and those who worked the sea. (There were "differences" of all sorts back then, between

the new and old, there are a million commercial fishing vessels out there, twice as many as in 1970, and able to catch almost twice as many fish each year as the ocean can sustainably produce.[3]

Now, hold on, you say, fish spawn more fish. That is true. But remember the ways these supertrawlers catch fish. Do you think they are carefully returning underage fish to the sea, like you could count on the lone fisherman to do? These new "harvesters" can reach into depths never before fished, and scientists play catch-up to make sure the new finds are okay to serve. One example of this is when, in haste to offer new products, orange roughy landed on the American menu. Later, scientists realized the fish lives nearly 150 years and does not reproduce until it is 30. In certain areas, the population has already collapsed.

race, class, sexual preference, and gender). I felt privileged to glimpse the lobstermen's experience and admired its authenticity. They caught their daily bread … for themselves and for their neighbors. A sense of admiration for the local lobstermen emanated from the summer people, similar to the way people used to feel about farmers. The lobstermen were trusted and respected; people were grateful for their hard work and wanted to protect their livelihood. My parents and grandparents would worry about the state of the lobster industry. Would there be enough for all the local pounds to stay open? I wish I could somehow share this with our children. The locals in the summer village we go to haven't owned the lobster pound for years.

My prize came one summer years ago, down at the pound. After sharing so many stories of the life of the lobster with me, the owner had saved something special just for me. It was a full lobster skin (lobsters shed their shells; hence, the soft-shell, hard-shell thing.) What made it particularly unique was that it was all in one piece. This was an amazing rarity … and he had kept it to give to me. My grandfather, the carver, built a special case to display the find.

Today the lobster skin sits on the top shelf of my children's playroom. Every few years, they ask me about it, and I get to tell them the story once again. Maybe with each telling I can pass on a glimmer of the gift of admiration for those neighbors who spend their lives catching our daily bread.

Another threat to our future fish capacity has to do with the food chain. As these supertrawlers sweep up the food eaten by the larger carnivorous fish, the ability to maintain populations at the higher levels of the chain is minimized.

Bycatch, unintended marine life caught in nets, has become a serious problem on all sorts of levels. One is the its sheer volume of waste, with almost one-fourth of all fished marine life being discarded each year because non-selective fishing methods capture non-targeted species.[4] Another problem is what can be caught in the nets: turtles, dolphins, and seals — sea animals that need our protection.

The National Marine Fisheries Service, in a report to Congress in 1999, concluded that 98 species in US waters are overfished and called the status of another 674 species "unknown." Marine scientists estimate that 60 to 70 percent of the world's commercial fisheries need urgent attention.[5]

The alternatives, fish farming and genetically engineered fish, have their own problems. Thankfully, some wonderful organizations are doing a great job of keeping us informed. I am just grateful they haven't suggested we write off seafood altogether, especially now that nutritionists have found further evidence of its health-providing characteristics. For a couple of years, we were asked to hold off on swordfish, but, according to Francine Stephens, new limits on catching Atlantic swordfish have resulted in the end of a two-year campaign for the ban on swordfish and released 70 chefs, grocery chains, and consumers from a pledge not to purchase swordfish. No problem, I think you'll agree — we can do our part if we know what that is. Just tell us what is necessary, and we will jump in.

> ## Shopping tip
>
> *"The Audubon Society's Living Oceans program has produced a wallet card, with categories from green (go ahead and eat) through yellow (caution, use your judgment) to red (stop – wait on this one.)"*

One of the best sources of information is the Audubon Society. Its Living Oceans program has produced a wallet card, with categories from green (go ahead and eat) through yellow (caution, use your judgment) to red (stop — wait on this one.) I downloaded it off the Audubon website **<www.audubon.org/campaign/lo>** and carry it in my wallet for quick reference at the grocery store. The program also has a wonderful chart giving full details on each fish — the background, population status, management, bycatch, habitat concerns, and alternatives. It is a wonderful resource, one that keeps changing and is updated every few months. In addition, Mercedes Lee, assistant director of the Living Oceans program, has written *Seafood Lover's Almanac*, a multifaceted book on the subject.

The Monterey Bay Aquarium in California **<www.mbayaq.org>** also offers a wallet card giving best choices, as well as a great deal of other information. The Seafood Choices Alliance, a new group formed in 2001, provides information to fishermen, chefs, and others on the environmental condition of the seafood industry. This group also produces a newsletter **<www.seafoodchoices.com>**.

If you forget to take your card to the grocery store, you can look for the relatively new eco-label, the first for fish products, of the Marine Stewardship Council (MSC). The council was originally formed in 1997 with Unilever (the world's largest buyer of seafood) and the World Wildlife Fund. Since 1999, it has operated independently in London. Its standards are based on the Code of Conduct for Responsible Fisheries, drawn up by the United Nations Food and Agriculture Organization.

EcoFish is a very dependable company that sells sustainable fish. For the past couple of years, I have stopped by their booth at the Natural Products Expo to have a chat and find out what

> ## Shopping tip
> *"If you forget to take your card to the grocery store, you can look for the relatively new eco-label, the first for fish products."*

else is happening in the world of fish. Since they were always very much on top of current news, studies, and trends, I expected their company to be large, with several employees tending to the "sustainable" portion of their business. With an advisory board that reads like an environmental fish-lovers' *Who's Who*, these guys are doing great business as well as providing consumers with a good, sustainable product. They even give 25 percent of pretax profits to support fish conservation efforts. At this year's Expo, I found out the truth: they are simply a young couple from New Hampshire who are trying to change the world, one fish dinner at a time. I get really excited when I learn about people who are truly dedicating their lives to good works.

Let's just go fish farming

Fish farming sounds like a great concept, but I am afraid we may have jumped in with both feet again, without taking enough precautions. Remember the Green Revolution? The idea was to alter plants so they would yield more, to feed more people. In a similar way, fish farming has been developed with the notion of supplementing our overtaxed ocean and lake fish. Sounds good. As a matter of fact, it could be very good, except that currently we are facing similar environmental consequences from fish farming. Thanks to an amazingly clear and concise study done by some leading environmentalists in aquaculture — Rebecca Goldburg and Matthew Elliot from Environmental Defense and Rosamund Naylor of Stanford University — we do have a picture of some of the environmental concerns.

Aquaculture has become big business on a global scale. Global production expanded at a rate of more than ten percent per year over the past decade, reaching 87 billion pounds (39.4 million tonnes) in 1998. While the US ranks third in national consumption of seafood and fourth in total fisheries catch, the country ranks eleventh in aquaculture production, with just 1.1 percent of global production by weight, or 1.6 percent by value. [6]

In terms of our dinner plates, aquaculture provides almost all of the catfish and trout consumed in the US, along with about half the shrimp and salmon.[7] If you ever wondered why catfish and salmon were sometimes priced as low as $3.99 a pound, it is because they are available from farms. Most (80 percent) of the US aquaculture production takes place in the South, particularly around the Mississippi Delta, which is the center of catfish farming. Channel catfish (Ictalurus punctatus), a freshwater species, accounts for more than 70 percent of farmed seafood fish in the US (by meat weight.)[8] The good news about catfish farming is that the farms tend to be smaller than those run by multinationals, which tend to stick to salmon farms.

Farming freshwater fish, such as catfish and tilapia, does take up a lot of land space and can add waste pollution to surrounding waterways. Aquaculture operations cover approximately 321,000 acres (130,000 ha) of fresh water in the US.[9] We are, however, encouraged to stick with these freshwater-farmed varieties, in part because they are herbivores and don't use up as much of our wild marine food sources as salmon do. Salmon, on the other hand, eat other animals, contributing to the depletion of small ocean fish.

Down on the salmon farms

The problems associated with fish farming seem to multiply when it comes to marine species, particularly salmon. First let's understand the different names of salmon so you know which to ask for. "Atlantic salmon" is the farmed version — there is no "Atlantic" wild version since, due to its low population, it is not sold in the US. There is some Pacific wild salmon, but both Atlantic and Pacific wild salmon are not recommended because, in part, of environmental degradation. But it, too, suffers from depletion of stocks. The one acceptable version is "Alaska wild salmon," as it is well regulated and sustained.

> ## Shopping tip
>
> *"The one acceptable version is "Alaska wild salmon," as it is well regulated and sustained."*

The whole explosion of fish farming seems to have started due to the lack of wild salmon. Bruce Barcott, writing for *Mother Jones*, states, "Modern fish farming traces its roots to Norway in the 1960s, when that nation's wild salmon stocks crashed due to overfishing, overdamming, acid rain, and development. Inspired by the success of Danish trout farmers, salmon cultivators found Norway's sheltered fjords ideal for farming salmon in ocean net pens ... the growth of fish farming (there became) marred by outbreaks of disease and parasites and the escape of millions of farm-bred salmon."[10]

The industry moved west to find new places to spawn, such as Scotland, Ireland, New Brunswick, then British Columbia and Alaska. All of those areas have experienced problems, except Alaska. That state had the foresight to keep the industry out. According to the Goldburg report, "Alaska — the state with the longest coastline — has altogether prohibited netpen and cage farming in coastal waters for the protection of native salmon populations and the human communities that depend upon them."[11]

Canada has become one of the largest salmon farming countries in the world, ranking fourth in worldwide production. Unfortunately, the country has suffered both wild and farmed casualties as they both try to coexist. "Canada's federal Department of Fisheries and Oceans (DFO), is charged with both promoting fish farming and conserving wild salmon runs. That dual mission has led the DFO to turn a blind eye to the environmental threat posed by the farms."[12]

Both British Columbia and New Brunswick have experienced their share of problems. On the East Coast, New Brunswick was directed to slaughter more than 1.2 million salmon in 1998 in an attempt to keep the disease Infectious Salmon Anemia (ISA) from spreading to other farms and into the wild. Unfortunately, in January 2001, ISA was found in a salmon farm in Maine, the first appearance in the US, and has since shown up in two more farms.[13]

British Columbia, a hotbed for salmon farming, has experienced myriad environmental problems, from gene sharing to waste management. One of the greatest environmental fears realized with salmon farming has been the mixing of farmed and wild species. While the industry defends its ability to keep the farmed version contained, scientists documented at least a quarter million Atlantic salmon escapes on the West Coast between 1987 and 1996, with another 350,000 escapes in 1997 alone.[14] According to the Canadian government, nearly 400,000 farm-raised Atlantics have escaped into British Columbia waters in the past decade. They weren't expected to be able to survive in the wild. However, by the summer of 2001, Atlantics had been found in 77 British Columbia rivers and streams.[15]

Beyond this form of biological pollution is the pollution from waste. From *Mother Jones:* "Typically, 15,000 to 50,000 fish share a single pen, and 8 to 10 pens operate on a single site. Since the pens are open to the surrounding water, any waste generated by the fish flushes into the local ecosystem. Farmers count on the tide to disperse netpen effluent, but the water often doesn't flush

"In 1997, four salmon netpens in Washington state discharged into Puget Sound 93 percent of the amount of "total suspended solids" produced by Seattle's sewage treatment plant."

it all away. A salmon farm of 200,000 fish releases an amount of fecal solids roughly equivalent to a town of 62,000 people."[16] How can fish create that much manure? They eat a lot. In 1997, four salmon netpens in Washington state discharged into Puget Sound 93 percent of the amount of "total suspended solids" produced by Seattle's sewage treatment plant.[17]

Again, as with factory farming, it seems to be a matter of size, with the big multinationals treating salmon like sardines, squeezing too many into spaces that are too small. Of course, what results from too many in too small a space is disease and subsequent chemical use, chemicals such as antibiotics, parasiticides (parasite-killing drugs), pesticides, hormones, anesthetics, various pigments, minerals, and vitamins.[18] Thankfully, antibiotics are not routinely served up in the fish feed, as on land factory farms. When administered, however, the drugs can be spread into waters beyond the immediate pens, with unknown effects on local ecosystems.

One of the biggest concerns surrounding salmon farming is that these fish are carnivores; they eat other fish. When raised in pens, salmon need to be fed, and their feed comes from the sea. Remember our earlier discussion of supertrawlers collecting everything they can? This is where a good percentage of that "bycatch" goes — right into fish feed. The big problem with this is that we are basically taking the food from the wild and bringing it to those in the pens, thus threatening the wild populations' survival. In addition, the quantity needed to feed the farm-raised species is enormous: about five kilograms of wild ocean fish, reduced to fish meal, are required to raise one kilogram of farmed ocean fish.[19]

For our own health purposes, farm-raised salmon tend to have less of the desired omega-3 fatty acids and, in order to mimic the wild version, dye is pumped through the fish. Remember, the wild version from Alaska is probably your best bet for salmon.

> **Shopping tip**
>
> *"For our own health purposes, farm-raised salmon tend to have less of the desired omega-3 fatty acids and, in order to mimic the wild version, dye is pumped through the fish. Remember, the wild version from Alaska is probably your best bet for salmon."*

Salmon shouldn't be the only farmed fish to receive such close investigation. Shrimp farming has caused plenty of devastation, particularly in countries such as Bangladesh, Indonesia, India, Thailand, and China. In Thailand, for example, annual production of giant tiger prawns has increased in the last decade from 900 tons to 277,000 tons.[20] Disease outbreaks, water demands, and requirements of feed and other resources have stretched some operations past their limit, leaving abandoned shrimp ponds exacting a heavy environmental toll.

Many problems are associated with aquaculture, and some wonderful people are working hard to find solutions, such as Integrated Pest Management for aquaculture, more secure pens for marine fisheries, and regulations that will limit quantities. These sustainable solutions are based on sound stewardship. But one development being heralded poses yet another threat. I bet you can guess.

Genetically modified fish, of course

At least 35 species of fish have been genetically engineered worldwide, although no transgenic fish products are commercially available yet. Thankfully, that makes this a short story. Short, only because the US Food and Drug Administration has yet to rule (although it may have by the time you read this, so check the Center for Food Safety website **<www.centerforfoodsafety.org>** for an update) on whether it will allow commercial sales of transgenic fish products.

Aqua Bounty Farms, a former subsidiary of A/F Protein, has applied to the FDA for permission to market genetically altered salmon. The company has devised technology to insert into an Atlantic salmon a growth-hormone gene from another fish, such as an ocean pout, so the salmon will grow more quickly. And grow, it does, reaching market weight in about 18 months, compared with the 24 to 30 months it normally takes to reach that size.[21]

Aqua Bounty president, Elliot Entis, said the company hoped to have regulatory approval from the US Food and Drug Administration by the summer of 2002 to sell its salmon eggs to commercial farmers. It also plans to apply for approval from Health Canada next spring.[22] Let's hope Aqua Bounty follows the path of two other companies, one in Scotland and another in New Zealand, who gave up in the face of negative press.

The biggest concern about genetically altered salmon is the danger of escape. We already know that, as much as industry has tried to avoid such a thing, large-scale escapes have become almost common. Two researchers from Purdue University, William Muir and Richard Howard, found frightening results could occur from such a release. Using a computer program and the Japanese medaka as an experimental model, the researchers plugged in data "to see what would happen when 60 transgenic fish were introduced into a population of 60,000 wild medaka. The results were disturbing. It took only 40 generations for the GM fish, whose size attracted mates more readily but whose offspring lacked survival skills, to drive the population to extinction. Muir and Howard called it the 'Trojan gene effect.'"[23]

Aqua Bounty's response has been to suggest they can provide sterile females. However, as diver/environmentalist Jean-Michael Cousteau argued, "Complete sterilization of all fish is simply not a reality. Nor is it likely to be. No company has stepped forward to guarantee 100 percent perfection in sterility. And nothing short of perfection is acceptable, for it only takes one well-endowed superfish in a population of wild salmon to start the process of decline."[24]

There are a couple of other problems. It seems these GE fish may have voracious appetites — wouldn't you if you had to grow that quickly? What that means, in terms of the increased demands for fish meal and the problems associated with that heavy marine toll, has rarely been discussed. It doesn't look good, particularly when we consider the influence of the industry on the regulators. Kent SeaFarms of San Diego received a $1.8 million grant from the US Department of Commerce to develop GE fish that grow more quickly, require less feed, and are more resistant.[25] Our tax dollars at work.

What about our health? Wouldn't you like to know if growth hormones in the fish you serve for dinner might affect you or your family? Since the FDA Center of Veterinary Medicine is charged with fish-farming regulations, human consumption evaluations aren't part of their purview. Those happen over at the USDA.

We could look to Aqua Bounty for reassurance. To quote Elliot Entis the company's president, "We are, I have to say, 100 percent certain that this is safe."[26]

Sounds fishy to me.

13

The Lowdown Behind the Labels

ECO-LABELS ARE OUR FRIENDS. They tell us the production methods used to grow our foods. Some are real (certified) and others are questionable. What do they mean and do they mean what they say?

"Organic" is a comforting term, one so comforting it was being used by producers who weren't actually using organic practices. Today, however, the US has national standards. But not all eco-labels focus on organic practices; some describe other production methods and values. Sometimes a little "Sherlock Holmes" helps ferret out the facts.

Eco-labels ... of approval

First, let's look at how environmental labeling came about. It began in Europe and did not start with food. Environmental labeling appears to have started with the German Blue Angel seal in the late 1970s, which was considered more of an award than a label of standards, denoting environmental excellence in certain manufactured products. Following on Germany's national program came Scandinavia's Nordic Swan, Canada's Environmental Choice, Japan's Ecomark, and the US Green Seal. These are not all public programs. Green Seal is privately managed by an independent, nonprofit organization, covering such product categories as household cleaners, paints, and fluorescent light bulbs.

The European Union's environmental label resembles a daisy and certifies appliances, such as refrigerators and washing machines, and household items, such as toilet paper. Canada's Environmental Choice eco-logo is on more than 1,400 approved products. A similar government-managed program in the US comes from the EPA using the EPA "energy star" and focuses on energy conservation in computer equipment.

Although these programs were the forerunners of eco-labels, they did not pertain to food. It is hard to identify the very first agricultural eco-label. In the late 1980s and early 1990s, Integrated Fruit Production (similar to today's Integrated Pest Management) was making its way across Europe, with more and more growers adopting "sustainable" practices. Although very strict production practices were highlighted, very little premium made its way back to growers, as consumer acceptance of the product as truly differentiated was minimal.

Around that time, I began working with University of Massachusetts Integrated Pest Management (IPM) scientists Craig Hollingsworth and Bill Coli and became aware of their work to bring an exciting new program, "Partners with Nature," to market. This program, developed by UMass and based on an IPM point system, was to become one of the first eco-labels in the US. Although it was a collaboration between the University of Massachusetts Extension, the Massachusetts Department of Food and Agriculture (MDFA), and the USDA, it seemed the majority of the project was handled by Bill and Craig. These two worked diligently to develop environmental standards for management of several different vegetable crops. Once the standards had been reviewed by colleagues and accepted, Bill and Craig needed to promote the concept and urge growers to voluntarily change their practices, submit exhaustive paper work, and become certified as part of Partners with Nature. No easy task; it was all so new at the time. The program would have benefited from successes in other parts of the country, had there been more, to help start the ball rolling.

To create enthusiasm around the concept, Bill, Craig, and Vicki Van Zee (another contributor in the world of sustainable agriculture) put together a conference (Growing Green, Selling Green) of manufacturers, consumers, growers, and anyone else who would be affected by the project, to discuss its virtues and barriers. It was a great success and added much-needed analysis at a point of infancy in the movement. They also conducted a New England–wide survey to determine the extent of grower and consumer interest. At the time, I had no idea how important their work was to become — what pioneers they were.

In its inaugural year, 40 growers were involved in the Partners with Nature program. Bill and Craig worked hard to put out brochures and signs at participating farms, and even a little print advertising. Their goal was to inform consumers, educate growers about IPM practices and promote IPM adoption. In 1998, they surveyed their growers and found 87 percent said the program provided them with a better understanding of IPM and 89 percent said it had helped them adopt more IPM practices. The Partners with Nature program was clearly becoming a model to improve environmental production. At conferences across the country, Bill and Craig were asked to speak on their experiences, and their papers were widely read by organizations initiating programs of their own.

Unfortunately, it seemed as though every year the funding from MDFA was questionable. Like politicians pulled away from their important work to campaign every four years, Bill and Craig were spending time each budget season justifying their fabulous program. In addition, the funding was never really enough. As more labels enter the market, project coordinators are becoming more aware of the necessity of an adequate eco-label marketing budget. Without it, consumers don't know enough about the labels to ask for them, and growers think consumers don't care, so they give up trying. The project's budget certainly did not cover substantial marketing.

> "If we can find out about our local eco-labels and purchase items meeting their standards, we send the signal to our state and federal authorities that we want these programs funded."

In the five years Partners with Nature was in existence, 89 growers were involved, but in the program's last year, it had only ten more than it had started with. This is a perfect example of how we, as consumers, could have made a difference. We might have been able to save Partners with Nature by asking for and buying its certified products. But who knew? Now we do. If we can find out about our local eco-labels and purchase items meeting their standards, we send the signal to our state and federal authorities that we want these programs funded.

Bill and Craig are still known for their pioneering efforts. If you bump into them, or any of our other eco-foods leaders, give 'em a high-five and say thanks for helping get labels off the ground!

Around the same time that Bill and Craig were starting their program, Stemilt Growers, a large fruit packer in Washington, began expanding on the European IFP program for its growers. This was one of the first where an actual label (with a ladybug and the words "Responsible Choice") was placed on the fruit itself. This seal differentiated the fruit and brought a $2 premium over an unlabeled box. Although the program has helped raise consumer awareness of environmental practices, it serves one company and is not available to other growers. The private nature of this program raises questions, although the standards are considered quite reputable.

Another program that started around the same time was at Wegmans Grocery store chain, based in Rochester, New York. The Wegman family learned of IPM practices and felt strongly enough about its potential to ask employee Bill Pool to initiate a program. Pool worked closely with Cornell entomologist Curt Petzoldt to develop IPM standards and contracted with Michigan's Comstock Foods, a canning company, to ensure their growers met IPM criteria. Where standards were met, the Cornell IPM logo was displayed on the can. Wegmans committed a great deal of resources to educate consumers and stand behind the program. Again, the product was sold by only one retail chain, but the standards were good and transparent.

The natural-food supermarket chain, Whole Foods, more recently considered developing a "sustainably grown" private label. The Whole Foods chain had been working on details of a plan to launch an IPM-based program for some of its products, but postponed it in the fall of 2001. The reason for holding off, according to company sources, is that the plan was developed prematurely, without input from some of the important producers, particularly those from the organic community. At this point, the Whole Foods label is on (or not on, depending how you look at it) the shelf.

Industry-led labeling requires particularly close examination. Some critics call these efforts "greenwashing" or, at least, an attempt by companies to promote themselves. ISO 14001, the environmental standards set up by industry similar to the ISO 9000 quality-control standards, have gotten little attention from the sustainable agriculture world, for this very reason. ISO 14001 is being picked up in other countries. New Zealand, Australia, Sweden, and Canada all have examples of farms developing their own plans for environmental management systems in accordance with the standards. Advocates of the standards point to global recognition of ISO as a virtue for international trade. At this point, there is a significant lack of awareness amongst the US agricultural community[1] about the standards.

Production practices

If eco-labels are all about standards, what do they mean? In the next chapters, we will review Integrated Pest Management (IPM) practices and organic practices. Most of the labels we have looked at so far are based on IPM systems, which have not received anywhere near the recognition level of organics, in part because the practices can vary to extremes. For that reason, organizations such as the Food Alliance and Protected Harvest have focused on setting and communicating their specific levels of practices. Before we talk more about these two groups, let's look at the newly arrived organic label. Forty-four different organic certification programs across the country (initiated by the California Certified Organic Growers) have been consolidated into one government-controlled organic label. Beginning October 2002, one of three different labels may appear on your grocery item: 100 percent Organic; Organic (95 percent); and Made with Organic (less than 95 percent organic content). To understand the meanings behind the terms, read Chapter 14.

> **"Forty-four different organic certification programs across the country (initiated by the California Certified Organic Growers) have been consolidated into one government-controlled organic label."**

Another production system that gets very little attention in the US but considerably more in Europe is Biodynamics, labeled as Demeter. Biodynamic agriculture (brought to us by Rudolph Steiner) emphasizes living soil, the delicate relationships within a whole farm system, and the balance of forces both seen and unseen. Biodynamic practices are in accord with the natural rhythms of nature, including those that have not been recognized by the scientific community as applicable. Practices tend to be conservation-oriented (such as soil quality improvements) as the system considers the health and vitality of the farm.

Very few people are aware of Biodynamic agriculture, in part because it is difficult to understand; it is not intuitive for our Cartesian minds. The system considers more than what we can analyze, so it is often disregarded. As a member of the Biodynamic Farmland Conservation Trust, I have struggled to understand the concepts. Most Biodynamic agriculture in this country is happening on community supported agriculture farms (see Chapter 20) a list of which is available through the Biodynamic Farming and Gardening Association **<www.biodynamics.com>**. You can also find a list of products that have received the Demeter seal, certifying application of the practices.

Who's who and how do we know?

Consumers Union has recently lent a hand to help us make decisions about eco-labels. Using its interactive website **<www.eco-labels.org>**, consumers can follow different paths to get to their label of choice, to review the official Consumers

Union opinion. A number of criteria are used to evaluate eco-labels: that the labels are meaningful and verifiable, consistent and clear, and transparent (all information used by the certifier is available to the public); that the certifier is independent and protected from conflict of interest; and that certification standards are developed with opportunities for public comment.

A few other organizations help us with Internet research on specific companies. One of my favorites is **<www.responsibleshopper.org>** from Working Assets and Co-op America; the Council of Economic Priorities at **<www.cepnyc.org>** is also a helpful tool; and **<www.corpwatch.org>**, Corpwatch — Holding Corporations Accountable, provides a variety of options to learn about the company behind the name.

One of the most important things to look for in the materials on an eco-label is the third-party certifier, meaning that whoever is chosen to certify should be independent of the project. Even in the case of Wegmans Grocery, the Cornell University entomologists were not the certifiers, because they developed the standards. This might have caused a conflict of interest, so they hired a number of IPM experts to check that the farms were applying the Cornell standards. This is very important; the third-party nature of the certifier is extremely critical.

One of those experts was Don Prostak, entomology professor emeritus from Rutgers University, who was later hired by Mothers & Others to certify the Core Values Northeast apple farms. Another early eco-label, Core Values was set up slightly differently. Instead of having a set of specific IPM standards for apples that all certified orchardists would use, Mothers & Others asked growers to submit orchard plans for improving their environmental practices, which would be approved or not, based on certain minimum criteria. No more or less legitimate than any other program, it is much needed within the apple industry.

Core Values Northeast is an interesting case study for another labeling issue. As the early eco-labels mature, some of them dissolve; others morph into a different entity all together. Mothers & Others was the lead environmental organization in the Core Values project, but after many years and huge contributions to improving our food system, it recently closed its doors. Interestingly, it was Mothers & Others for a

WEBSITE WEBSITE WEBSITE

> ### Shopping tip
>
> *"One of the most important things to look for in the materials on an eco-label is the third-party certifier, meaning that whoever is chosen to certify should be independent of the project."*

Liveable Planet (their first name) that brought actress Meryl Streep to speak out against the pesticide Alar on apples. The apple industry was furious, and yet that same organization helped growers who did want to improve their environmental behavior find a premium at the market through Core Values.

Like any other eco-label, Core Values has struggled to gain recognition from consumers, but it continues to function. Having no other partners, Core Values was in need of a home. Today the Conservation Law Foundation in Boston (another unexpected hero in the food arena) has taken it on. However, instead of taxing the foundation with the need for extensive marketing support, there is now some discussion of merging Core Values with another label program.

Food Alliance approved

One of the most successful label programs is on the West Coast. The Food Alliance is doing one thing very, very well: communicating. They let consumers know all about their certified farmers via their website and through point-of-purchase display materials at supermarkets and farmers' markets. Their funding seems solid, in part because their results are clearly positive. The big drawback, until recently, has been their fairly small regional coverage. You are lucky if you live in the Northwest because you will see the labels on fruits, vegetables, jams and jellies, cheeses and milk, meats, wheat, and wines in more than 500 retail outlets. (Remember, if your market does not already stock them, request Food Alliance-approved products from your grocery store manager.)

> "One of the most successful label programs is on the West Coast. The Food Alliance lets consumers know all about their certified farmers via their website and through point-of-purchase display materials at supermarkets and farmers' markets."

In October 2000, the Food Alliance expanded into Minnesota under the auspices of the Midwest Food Alliance. Food Choices was the original name of the collaboration between the Land Stewardship Project, the Organic Alliance, and the Wisconsin-based Cooperative Development Services. Director Jim Ennis reviewed the research, the experiences of other programs, and the potential of his market area, and decided to stick with a winner. The Food Alliance had already been successful in the Northwest, and Food Choices hoped to duplicate the program in their area.

What does it really mean to be a Food Alliance farm? Jonathan Moscatello, agriculture program manager, gave a great synopsis of the process for *Grist* magazine last spring: "First, the producers that wish to become Food Alliance-approved send in a detailed application that explicitly outlines their practices. Then a third-party inspector visits the farm or ranch for an on-site evaluation using commodity-specific evaluation criteria (we have specific guidelines for over 200 commodities). The inspector then submits the evaluation to me, and if the operation has achieved a 70 percent score or better in all categories, it becomes eligible to market its product using our Food Alliance-approved label."[2]

When standards are involved, there always seems to be some level of discussion about rigor. Do the certifying criteria expect too much or too little of growers? Do they raise the bar on environmental quality so high that too few growers can reach it or can anyone, with a little modification, achieve the minimal standards?

Protected Harvest

These tricky questions were posed often during the development of the Protected Harvest program. Its standards were developed through a collaboration of the World Wildlife Fund, the Wisconsin Potato and Vegetable Growers Association, and the University of Wisconsin at Madison, with the goal of environmental improvement of potato-growing practices. Potatoes are one of the most heavily sprayed crops, although they have little pesticide residue, since they grow underground. In the early 1980s the highly toxic insecticide aldicarb was detected regularly in the region's drinking water,[3] bringing the need for less chemical-dependent pest management systems to the forefront.

Dean Zeulegar of the WPVGA, representing 250 growers with more than 80,000 acres of potatoes, went to the World Wildlife Fund to initiate discussions about an IPM-based solution. What ensued was a long process of working out the goals and details of what has become a highly successful project. This eco-label is unusual because of the duration of planning, the level of expertise, and the commitment of the triad of collaborators to endure an exhaustive search for the highest quality standards. With the help of Chuck Benbrook, these bio-intensive IPM practices include limits on toxicity units of pesticides and a total exclusion list for 12 pesticides. The program has been highly successful in reducing the use of targeted pesticides and those with greatest toxicity levels.

Okay, I must come clean: this is the program I became enmeshed in during the last year. I worked with these wonderful growers, academics, and environmentalists on ways to best communicate with consumers. Extensive research on other labels

Got a cold?
Try "Healthy Grown" potato soup

This soup recipe is one I made up recently when I was in the early stages of a cold. You know that feeling — all achey and uncomfortable, the nose alternately filling and draining, the throat raw and battered? I was in that stage when faced with either a trip to the grocery store or some creative handling of some basics I had at home — a bag of "Healthy Grown" potatoes, a can of organic tomatoes in the cabinet, a wedge of leftover onion in the refrigerator, some red lentils left in the bean jar, garlic, and gingerroot. The grocery store was clearly more than I could handle, so here is what I did:

Saute in a tablespoon of olive oil:
$^1/_4$–$^1/_2$ onion
3–4 garlic cloves, chopped.

Add:

3–4 cups of antibiotic-free chicken broth (or water, if nothing else is around)
1 cup of red lentils, washed and picked over
2" cube of gingerroot, chopped.
Bring to a boil and simmer for about 30 minutes.
Add a few potatoes, cut into cubes, and the can of tomatoes.
Continue to simmer for another 15 minutes.

When I made this, I threw in a tablespoon of powdered ginger for the last five minutes. It gave the soup a very strong ginger flavor, but it worked very nicely on the achey, cold feeling. The combination of ginger and garlic is supposed to be good for your immune system. I am not an herbalist, but it certainly tasted good and seemed to clear out my head a bit. Now that I think of it, that cold never did really amount to much. Maybe the soup helped more than I thought. Try it!

reinforced in my mind the superior quality of the standards. So although I am a bit biased, I also have the benefit of seeing first-hand the level of commitment and dedication of these folks. But don't depend on me. The real test came when Jeff Dlott, the behind-the-scenes ringleader, sought potential board members for Protected Harvest. The response was immediate and impressive. If you question my opinion, check out the individuals who have agreed to be actively involved with the program (by checking out the website **<www.protectedharvest.org>**). They read like a *Who's Who* in environmental heroes!

There were several heroes on this project. Sarah Lynch from the World Wildlife Fund helped keep the project front and center at that organization. But the real heroes are the people you will never read about: Deana Sexson and Kit Schmidt from UWM; Randy Duckworth, Mike Carter, Stacey Steckbauer, and Karen Walters from the WPVGA; and all the growers. These are the people who showed up at the grueling day-long meetings to iron out much of the minutiae. There are heroes like these on all projects (I just happen to know this gang), and many won't make it to the limelight.

Labeling ... other stuff

From bananas and coffee to fish and wood, more and more environmentally conscious programs are working to let you know what has been produced with the Earth in mind. You read about the Rainforest Alliance in Chapter 8. Their labels range from the ECO-OK bananas and coffees to Smart Voyager, the eco-label for sustainable tourism.

The forest has also been an arena for eco-labeling efforts. The Forest Stewardship Council, developed with a number of supporters, including the World Wildlife Fund, works with Smart Wood, a labeling program initially sponsored by the Rainforest Alliance. Both are legitimate international programs. Smart Wood has impressive standards, yet minimal consumer awareness. A big coup for its efforts came a few years ago when Home Depot agreed to carry certified product. Unfortunately, consumers have not found their way to the certified woods as much as some had hoped. So if you are building something, ask for their certified product!

> ### Shopping tip
> "Rainforest Alliance labels range from the ECO-OK bananas and coffees to Smart Voyager, the eco-label for sustainable tourism."

WEBSITE

The Marine Stewardship Council, based on the model of the Forest Stewardship Council and also led by World Wildlife Fund, has had its growing pains due to the controversy surrounding a major initial partner, Unilever, one of the largest international buyers of fish. Unilever controls 20–25 percent of the European and North American frozen white fish market, and it has pledged to obtain all of its seafood products from sustainable sources by 2005.[4] If the standards were minimal and Unilever controlled their development, it would certainly be a case for greenwashing. However, once again the standards are impressive, and the Marine Stewardship Council is clearly its own non-profit organization, working to certify fisheries all over the world.

How can we, as consumers, know whether or not a program is legitimate? Do we immediately assume it is not if a corporate entity is involved? That should not be a base criteria, as proven by the case of the Marine Stewardship Council. We have seen with Wegmans and (almost) Whole Foods that a retailer-led program may be credible, especially when a land grant university is involved. Does this mean that when a large and highly respected environmental organization is a partner, it automatically spells success? Not according to the Consumers Union. The Nature Conservancy and the World Wildlife Fund both lend their logos to products in exchange for donations. When you buy a certain product, X percentage will go to support the environmental group. It is considered a helpful way for the environmental organization to raise much-needed funds that may eventually go into developing standards for some other program. But it is also confusing to buyers. These two organizations, for example, have been and continue to be involved in developing tough environmental standards and market incentive programs, and have been essential collaborators in the sustainable agriculture movement.

Back to fish, Salmon Safe is a non-profit affiliate of the Pacific Rivers Council, one of the leading US fish conservation programs. Launched in 1997, Salmon Safe approves labels on agricultural products that meet certain production criteria that reduce chemical runoff in areas where salmon spawn. A serious issue in the Northwest, Salmon Safe gives consumers the power to contribute to the solution by buying approved foods and drinks.

> **Shopping tip**
>
> *"Launched in 1997, Salmon Safe approves labels on agricultural products that meet certain production criteria that reduce chemical runoff in areas where salmon spawn."*

Shopping tip

"One of the newest programs is the Free-Farmed Certification Program, offering a set of animal husbandry standards that ensure access to clean and sufficient food and water, and a safe and healthful living environment. With a quick check at <www.eco-labels.org>, we can find the Consumers Union thumbs-up approval of the program."

What about dolphin-safe, you may be wondering. Originally, Earth Island Institute helped to save the day (or the dolphins) by bringing much-needed attention to the situation. Providing one of the few labels clearly recognized by most consumers, this program is now administered by the government and labels tuna caught without the use of certain nets that can trap and kill dolphins in areas where tuna and dolphins swim together. It also ensures regular inspection of fishing boats in these areas.[5] Another lesser-known and more recent project brought to attention by Earth Island Institute is the issue of endangered turtles being killed by shrimp nets. Similar to the dolphin-safe program, shrimp fishermen will have the opportunity to become certified as turtle-safe.

One of the newest programs is the Free-Farmed Certification Program, offering a set of animal husbandry standards that ensure access to clean and sufficient food and water, and a safe and healthful living environment. Developed by the American Humane Association, the certification can be found on meat, dairy, and poultry products. With a quick check at **<www.eco-labels.org>**, we can find the Consumers Union thumbs-up approval of the program.

In recent years, discussions have been brewing at sustainable agriculture conferences about whether or not so many labels confuse the consumer. I have always advocated for the more, the better. There is so much these different organizations, different production practices, or different species-saving groups do for our Earth. I am just grateful for them all. Remember, though, now it is our turn. With every purchase, we do our part.

WEBSITE

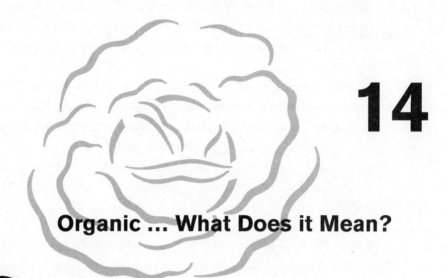

Organic ... What Does it Mean?

CONTROVERSIAL AS IT CAN BE IN SOME CIRCLES, organic production is one of the best forms of agriculture we've got. And, thanks to 275,603 citizen comments on the first proposal for national organic standards, and 40,774 on the second, we now have federal regulations intended to weed out the guys who say they're following organic practices but are not.

This chapter is devoted to the one method of farming that, to date, addresses our most fundamental concerns: the use of pesticides, genetically altered ingredients, growth hormones and (subsequently) increased antibiotics, sewage sludge, and irradiation. The method has an understandable definition, and it comes to us under certification by way of a national label.

Organic: what does it mean?

What does "organic" really mean? The definition passed by the National Organic Standards Board at its April 1995 meeting and so far upheld is:

> Organic agriculture is an ecological production management system that promotes and enhances biodiversity, biological cycles, and soil biological activity. It is based

on minimal use of off-farm inputs and on management practices that restore, maintain, and enhance ecological harmony.

"Organic" is a labeling term that denotes products produced under the authority of the Organic Foods Production Act. The principal guidelines for organic production are to use materials and practices that enhance the ecological balance of natural systems and that integrate the parts of the farming system into an ecological whole.

Organic agriculture practices cannot ensure that products are completely free of residues; however, methods are used to minimize pollution from air, soil, and water.

Organic food handlers, processors, and retailers adhere to standards that maintain the integrity of organic agricultural products. The primary goal of organic agriculture is to optimize the health and productivity of interdependent communities of soil life, plants, animals, and people.[1]

That helps, but what does it really *mean*? In a wonderful interview in *Acres USA*, titled "The True Meaning of 'Organic,'" organic farmer and director of the Leopold Center Fred Kirschenmann says, "In organic agriculture, you are trying to cooperate with nature, not subdue nature ... Fundamentally, the idea is — as the word organic itself implies — to integrate various parts into a whole living organism."[2] Author and organic advocate Grace Gershuny says, "First and foremost, the organic world view replaces the notion of domination with one of cooperation."[3]

This concept of working *with* versus *against* comes through loud and clear in the following quote from Justus von Liebig, the German chemist credited with leading the way into chemical agriculture by proving that plants could take up simple compounds of nitrogen, phosphorus, and potassium and convert them into protein and carbohydrates. Looking back on his life and work, he said, in 1865, "I have sinned against the wisdom of the creator and, justly, I have been punished. I wanted to improve his work because, in My blindness, I believed that a link in the astonishing chain of laws that govern and constantly renew life on the surface of the Earth had been forgotten. It seemed to me that weak and insignificant man had to redress his oversight."[4]

Typically assigned the honor of opening the doors to organic agriculture are scientists Sir Albert Howard and Lady Eve Balfour who, in the 1940s, wrote about the interrelationship of soils, plants, animals, and people. J.I. Rodale is then credited with popularizing the methods in his *Organic Farming and Gardening* magazine. At about the same time, however, chemical agriculture was taking off as "leftovers" from a new industry, initiated for the World Wars, found a new home — our farmers' fields. It was not until the 1960s that organic agriculture took off again, thanks to that bold and brave biologist, Rachel Carson. Then a ragtag bunch of hippies took off to communes in California to raise foods. Those smart young people were out to find a solution, and many of them did. Certainly there were a lot more folks besides the hippies who were frustrated with the chemical approach and who wanted to see "life" brimming on their farms. Many of these people began a revolution toward sustainability. The world of Integrated Pest Management was making its way onto the fields. The importance of "ecology" was becoming part of agricultural discussions. All the while, organic production was being practiced; Europe was beginning to demand organic products; and items referred to as organic began to appear in health food stores across the country.

> "In 1989, the television program 60 Minutes aired an exposé on the dangers of Alar, a chemical used by the apple industry to reduce early dropping of the fruit. All of a sudden, the public wanted chemical-free food, and they wanted it now …"

Then in 1989, the television program *60 Minutes* aired an exposé on the dangers of Alar, a chemical used by the apple industry to reduce early dropping of the fruit. All of a sudden, the public wanted chemical-free food, and they wanted it now … for a short time. As happens in response to many media stories, our awareness spiked and then slowly over time, the pressure waned and people got back to their everyday lives. The demand shot up, then slowed, yet never totally receded.

Since then, the organic industry has been growing at a rate of 20 percent every year. (Conventional grocery sales increase approximately 3 percent each year.) Sales of organic products in 2000 were nearly $7.7 billion, still small compared with $400 billion in the food industry overall. Organics got big … and no surprise, the big multinational food companies want a piece of that pie.

Let's play fair

At the same time that sales were increasing in North America, demands for organically produced products were intensifying very quickly in Europe. Consistency of standards across borders began the initial push for industry-wide parity. As Fred Kirschenmann said, "We originally got into the certification business because, back 20 years ago when we started it, there wasn't any certification program in the United States that met the requirements in Europe. Some of our growers and one of the companies that we were selling grain to wanted to export some of the product into Europe. We just decided that we would start a program that would meet the requirements in Europe. Once we got into certification, it became clear to me that certification was one of the ways of trying to keep the organic system pure."[5]

This seems consistent with some of the stories I have heard about the early days of organic standards from Judy Gillan. Judy was one of those instrumental in developing consistent production language and in founding the Organic Foods Production Association of North America, the precursor to today's Organic Trade Association, the industry association that promotes and protects the integrity of organic standards.

Since there was little consensus at that time, the verification process started out fragmented. The California Certified Organic Farmers offered the first organic certification in 1973, soon followed by other certification organizations in other regions of the country. By 1985, at least 12 separate entities offered organic certification.[6] By the time the national organic standards were announced in December 2000, 44 private or public organizations were certifying farms using different production practices under the same term: "organic."

With little uniformity in place and demand growing, both consumers and growers wanted to clear up the confusion emanating from the organic world. To that end, the Organic Foods Production Act was born within the 1990 Farm Bill. As part of the Act, the National Organic Program was formed to establish organic standards and oversee mandatory certification. The USDA acts as the overseer of the program, and states or private organizations administer it.

As part of the directive, the USDA was required to base the certification program on the recommendations of a 15-member National Organics Standards Board (NOSB) that includes four farmers, two processors, one retailer, one scientist, three consumer advocates, three environmentalists, and one certifying agent. In 1995, the group released the definition of organics provided at the beginning of this chapter. The board called for an unprecedented amount of information to help form their recommendations. In addition to their input, the USDA also reviewed the existing certification programs and those from other countries. In the end, the first set of proposed rules looked very little like the work from the NOSB. In December 1997, the first set of rules was published and received an amazing 275,603 public comments, decrying the proposed rules.

The overall sentiment of the industry and concerned consumers was summed up by final comments from Peter Hoffman, a board member of the Chef's

Collaborative and organic food advocate in a *New York Times* Op-Ed piece: "The Agriculture Department's new guidelines don't need minor tweaking or revision. They need to be scrapped and rewritten in accordance with the original recommendations by the National Standards Board — an approach that considers the health of all living things along the food chain and tells consumers the truth about what they're buying."[7] Clearly, the USDA had been sent back to the drawing board.

Around that time, Jack Kittredge of the Northeast Organic Farming Association gave a seminar at the University of Massachusetts about the standards. He explained about the "Big Three" practices allowed by the proposed standards and considered the worst of all the recommendations: genetically modified organisms (GMOs), sewage sludge, and irradiation.

Sewage sludge, or reprocessed sewage from human and industrial waste, is used in conventional farming, but has been identified as a potential source of heavy metals. The organic community has always rejected the use of sludge on fields, as plants may potentially take up the contaminants from the soil, which then show up in our foodstuffs. Apparently, using sewage sludge in fertilizer solves some economic problems. In a MacNeil/Lehrer Newshour panel discussion, the issue of sludge was discussed and identified as some people's answer to what to do with the billion tons of sewage cities generate each year. As the PBS reporter concluded, "Pouring it on oceans is illegal. Dumping it into landfills is expensive. The technical director of Orange County, California's Sanitation District says the county saves $10 per ton recycling its 180,000 tons of sludge onto crop lands."[8] What will they think of dumping on our dinner next?

The final of the Big Three issues answers that question. They can dump just about anything if they then turn around and zap it full of radiation, killing all the bad — and good — stuff it contains. (Irradiation was discussed in Chapter 9.) Well, let's not keep us in suspense any longer — all three of these concerns were eliminated in the final proposal. Phew! There were a number of other concerns during the first go-around, such as animals being labeled organic yet being fed only 80 percent organic feed, and animal confinement.

On December 21, 2000, nine months after a second proposed rule was submitted, the USDA released its much-improved final version of national organic standards. The core of the standards is the Farm Plan and Handling Plan, where producers and processors prove to certifiers that they can apply not only the standards but principles of organic agriculture. There is also a list of allowed synthetic and prohibited natural substances, such as those used for processing or disinfecting services, that might come in contact with the food. Some organic advocates are concerned the list is not tight enough in the area of allowable processing ingredients. In general, we can feel confident that there are no allowable synthetic pesticides or fertilizers. In response to the initial protests, irradiation, sewage sludge, and GMOs are not allowed. Producers can add other labels (eco or otherwise). Organic animals are to be fed 100 percent organic grain and will not receive regular feedings of antibiotics or growth hormones. There were other issues as well, and critics felt the standards fell short. In general, both sides lost a little and ultimately, we consumers won a lot. Now we can at least attempt to know consistently what organic means.

It is really no surprise that defining organic agriculture would be so difficult — the method goes much deeper than rules can express. "Organic food is not just about a product; it is a philosophy in which the process of production is as important as the final result. Organic growers rightly believe that a farm is a diverse ecosystem, that soil is a living organism to be nurtured, and that farming practices need to be concerned about the long-term health of workers, consumers, the surrounding water supply, and the animals living within the habitat."[9] Trying to wrestle this value system down onto paper is hard enough. Now try to turn it into rules with little room for personal interpretation. It sounds like organized religion trying to interpret spirituality. At some point, we have to make our own decisions, based on all we can understand. As John Ikerd of the University of Missouri put it, "You can't write standards for how you treat your neighbor down the road or for a commitment to community or concern for maintaining the health of the soil."[10]

> "Organic food is not just about a product; it is a philosophy in which the process of production is as important as the final result."

So now we have organic standards. The final rule went into affect on April 21, 2001, and will be fully implemented on October 21, 2002. According to the Organic Trade Association, "The word 'organic' on US products will mean that the ingredients and production methods have been verified by an accredited certification agency as meeting or exceeding USDA standards for organic production."[11] Growers (who make over $5,000 a year) will submit farm plans and records and undergo periodic farm inspections for soil and water tests. Handlers or anyone involved with the direct processing of organic products will also be certified.

The growth of organics

What about our neighbors to the North? Canadians have witnessed a similar explosion in organic products, thanks in part to major grocery chains, particularly Loblaws. Not only has Loblaws been building natural-foods sections into their stores, they have created a private label, President's Choice Organics, with 25 current products and 200 more in the offing. Wild Oats Markets acquired Capers stores in British Columbia, with further openings anticipated, and Whole Foods Market expects to open ten of its stores throughout the provinces over the next few years.

> "Not only has Loblaws been building natural-foods sections into their stores, they have created a private label, President's Choice Organics, with 25 current products and 200 more in the offing."

Canadian acreage devoted to organics is climbing, with 1.3 percent of total cropland, but still only 0.8 percent of the total number of farms in Canada. According to a recent article in the *Ottawa Citizen*, "Since 1990, the organic food industry has grown by 20 percent a year, and that growth has not kept pace with demand. In Ontario, there is a waiting list for stores that want to sell organic milk, but not enough dairies to supply them, said Larry Lenhardt, head of the Organic Crop Producers and Processors (OCPP), a certification agency based in Lindsay, Ontario."[12]

Organic standards were developed in Canada earlier than in the US, but, like other standards under Canada's National Standards System, they remain voluntary. This does not mean growers cannot certify their practices; they simply receive that certification from a third party, like the OCPP. Currently, Canada is in the process of revising its standards to be more consistent with those in the US and Europe.

Europe, looking at trade, had reached consensus on a definition of organic back in 1993. So, not surprisingly, they are a little ahead of the game. According to a World Watch report in the summer of 2001, "In Europe, organic foods now account for 3–5 percent of sales ... Europeans are spending nearly $10 billion on organic products each year."[13] And in terms of acreage, "The total area of farmland devoted to cultivating organic crops has grown to an estimated 11.5 million hectares — roughly the size of Cuba ... In Western Europe, organic area has ballooned 35-fold since 1985 — increasing roughly 30 percent each year ... In Austria, the organic share has reached 10 percent ... Denmark has set a 50 percent organic (acreage) target by 2012 ... In the United Kingdom, the proposed Organic Food and Farming Targets Bill (that has already been through one rejection) would require that by

2010 not less than 30 percent of agricultural land in England, Wales, and Northern Ireland is certified organic or in conversion, and not less than 20 percent by volume of food consumed is organic."[14]

In the US, acreage devoted to organic farming is still less than 0.2 percent of the cropland, but the numbers are increasing rapidly, with a 47 percent increase from 1995 to 1997. The good news continues: the number of certified organic farms and acres in the US almost doubled since 1995 while the total number of farms and acres decreased over the same time period.[15]

Another piece of good news is that organic agriculture seems to have attracted a different group of farmers. While the average age of a conventional farmer is mid-fifties, organic farmers tend to be in their mid-forties. In terms of education, 32 percent of certified organic farmers have completed college, and 18 percent hold graduate degrees.[16] That is not a big surprise, with so much of the practice demanding that highly educated, "ecologically sound" decisions be made from minute to minute. Whether working to balance the beneficial insects with those that cause damage, rotating crops, monitoring compost decomposition rates for soil fertility, or mapping potential drift from neighboring GMO-planted fields, organic farmers have a lot on their minds.

> "Organic agriculture seems to have attracted a different group of farmers. While the average age of a conventional farmer is mid-fifties, organic farmers tend to be in their mid-forties."

Is this why organic products cost so much more? The intricacies are certainly part of the costs, but the biggest factor in the added expense is the labor, particularly for weeding. Remember, organic farmers cannot use chemical herbicides, the number one pesticide used by conventional agriculture. So, what to do? Obviously, if a farm is hundreds or thousands of acres, the farmer cannot hand-weed the rows, but must rely on more mechanical cultivation. Most small organic growers hire hand-weeders, and that can get very costly. Think of how long it takes you to do your own garden, then imagine a huge field!

The price factor is often turned into a snide comment by naysayers, who refer to organics as "yuppie food." Interestingly, it is not the wealthy baby boomers alone who buy organics; it seems to be an equal opportunity choice. But it will surely take a greater share of the weekly grocery tab for some.

There are plenty of naysayers out there, but none can rival the organic industry's most verbal adversaries: Dennis Avery and his son, Alex. I don't really understand their motivation, except, of course, that it may be financial. Dennis Avery runs the

Center for Global Food Issues, a project of the Hudson Institute funded by such companies as Monsanto, Dow, and Eli Lilly. The Averys are not only aggressive in the media and in their own writing, but they have been accused of misquoting and fabricating some of their research. They play on fears that might make sense but are unfounded, such as "more potential for bacteria contamination." They referred to findings by the US Centers for Disease Control, but the CDC subsequently refuted any such studies. One of the Averys' favorite statements is that crop yields are so low with organic agriculture that wild habitat would be significantly affected by wholesale conversion. In a debate with Rebecca Goldburg from the Union of Concerned Scientists, he actually used the numbers, "55 to 60 percent of conventional yields."[17] In this case, it appears he was just plain wrong.

More and more studies have been emerging to indicate that organics can produce nearly the same yields as conventional agriculture. As a matter of fact, Bill Liebhardt at the University of California at Davis did a review of the literature and found that "for a total of 154 growing seasons for different crops, grown in different parts of this country on both rain-fed and irrigated land, organic production yielded 95 percent of crops grown under conventional high-input conditions."[18]

Are the Averys the only naysayers? Certainly not. As one might imagine, the conventional grocery industry is not so happy. In December 2001, when the revised rules were announced, the National Food Processors Association asked the USDA to require that organic labels include a statement saying the products are no more safe or nutritious than conventional foods. In the end, the USDA did not require the disclaimer but did modify the label design by dropping the traditional USDA shield and eliminating "certified" from the seal.[19] The Grocery Manufacturers Association also opposed many aspects of the standards, particularly those related to the consumer's perception of food safety. Many say this is why former Agriculture Secretary Dan Glickman kept referring to the seal as "a marketing tool" that did not imply organic foods are either safer or more nutritious.

I understand that not enough studies have been done to attribute either of these benefits to organic products. Some are trickling in ... one study here, another there, but too premature to be definitive. As stated in the *US News & World Report*, "For consumers worried about diet and health, the big difference is that organic foods are virtually free of the synthetic chemicals found in regular produce. The fruits and vegetables in a typical produce aisle may contain anywhere from one to a half-dozen pesticide residues ... In large doses, many of these chemicals can cause cancer, nervous system damage, and other ills. The risks, if any, of the traces found in your salad and fruit bowls are not known. Weighing the threat is especially tough when it comes to children, whose developing bodies may be more vulnerable and who eat large amounts of fruits and vegetables."[20] It may not be official to say organically grown foods are more nutritious and safe, but as a mom, I know one thing. While the jury is out, I will try to stick with organics.

> "It may not be official to say organically grown foods are more nutritious and safe, but as a mom, I know one thing. While the jury is out, I will try to stick with organics.

Who will win this game?

There is a buzz in the organic industry and today it is not specifically about the standards. It is about an emerging rift amongst individuals in the organics industry. As some of the pioneering organic products move into sales figures usually reserved for conventional items, some fear the loss of the original intention. Today, familiar organic brands are owned by big business. Stonyfield Farm is now owned by Danone; Cascadian Farm is owned by General Mills; Vermont's Organic Cow is owned by Horizon Organic Dairy. Clearly, consolidation is not left only to the conventional grocery industry. Today five giant farms control half of California's $400 million organic produce market.[21]

Many of the big organic businesses are owned by the movement's originators, who have come to believe this outcome as inevitable, a success in its own right. Gene Kahn, who started Cascadian Farms years ago as a cooperative, expressed this sentiment: "You have a choice of getting sad about all that or moving on. We tried hard to build a cooperative community and a local food system, but at the end of the day it wasn't successful. This is just lunch for most people. Just lunch. We can call it sacred, we can talk about communion, but it's just lunch."[22] I guess I don't believe that, nor do I believe he did, either, when he started out. But he is not alone. Myra Goodman, who founded Earthbound 17 years ago and now markets its products in all 50 states, said "We're pushing organics where it hasn't gone before ... The supermarkets around the country wouldn't be carrying organics if the whole supply was a bunch of small growers."[23]

If they have to play by rules anyway, what is wrong with industrial organic agriculture? Many of these mega-organic farms are also converting otherwise pesticide-laden land to fields of fertility. They still have to play by the rules, and now the rules are clear: no synthetic fertilizers, pesticides, GMOs, antibiotics, sewage sludge, irradiation, etc. This is a good thing.

Michael Pollan wrote of his experience with the new big business controversy. "My journey through the changing world of organic food has cured me of my naive supermarket pastoralism, but it hasn't put me off my organic feed. I still fill my cart with the stuff. The science might still be sketchy, but common sense tells me organic is better food — better, anyway, than the kind grown with organophosphates, with antibiotics and growth hormones, with cadmium and lead and arsenic (the EPA permits the use of toxic waste in fertilizers), with sewage sludge and animal feed made from ground-up bits of other animals as well as their own manure. Very likely it's better for me and my family, and

> "Now the rules are clear: no synthetic fertilizers, pesticides, GMOs, antibiotics, sewage sludge, irradiation, etc. This is a good thing."

unquestionably it is better for the environment. For even if only 1 percent of the chemical pesticides sprayed by American farmers end up as residue in our food, the other 99 percent are going into the environment — which is to say, into our drinking water, into our rivers, into the air that farmers and their neighbors breathe. By now it makes little sense to distinguish the health of the individual from that of the environment."[24]

Can't we all play?

Fred Kirschenmann of the Leopold Center usually has an important contribution. In an article in *Acres USA*, he suggests, "It seems like the goal of the industry in the 'mainstream' organic market is to put a certified organic product in place of every conventional product … the effort ought to be not to replace every conventional product with a certified organic product, but to create a whole new food system with a diverse set of products … We ought to be doing a whole range of other crops to create markets for the diverse crops that farmers need to have a diverse crop rotation."[25] This out-of-the box idea is what we need — increasing diversity beyond the products and into the realm of solutions.

Grace Gershuny is also good for a solution: "Large agribusiness companies can conceivably convert millions of acres of farmland to organic production, destined for processed products such as breakfast burritos, at the same time that activists continue promoting the virtues of buying locally grown foods and joining community-supported agriculture farms. The two are not mutually exclusive, and the opportunity to buy organic products in familiar places like supermarkets and even convenience stores may initiate many people, who are unlikely to venture into health food stores, into greater awareness of how their food is produced."[26] Grace's suggestion seems consistent with others I have heard in the industry. Both avenues result in comparatively good news. "Ultimately, two complementary markets for organic products may develop: the industrial organic stream, which services major supermarkets and food manufacturers, and the local and regional organic stream, which maintains a strong connection to consumers."[27] This seems inevitable.

Who will win this game? It seems like we *all* will.

15

What Does IPM Mean?
Control Freaks in the Field

SOME FARMERS (AND SCIENTISTS) INSIST WE JUST CAN'T GROW EVERYTHING organic. IPM takes the best and the least of the worst to bring us the fruits of a lot of labor. This chapter describes the methods used as part of Integrated Pest Management (IPM). IPM is a broad name for growing practices that lessen environmental impacts. Depending on the level or point in the continuum, some people suggest IPM sits somewhere between organic and conventional. It, too, has its share of controversy; many say it does not go far enough, while others who say their environmental conditions won't support organic feel they should be respected for making extra efforts. IPM has been accepted by the USDA as a viable alternative to conventional growing, with many of our tax dollars going to research and education in the field. Many of the eco-label programs discussed in Chapter 9 use IPM production practices as the basis of their standards. So what does it mean?

It may not work so well in your personal relationships, but being an IPM control freak in the field is certainly better than spraying all sorts of chemicals by the calendar. For many years, the "silver bullet" pesticides were scheduled and delivered whether a pest was lunching in the fields or not. As we learned in Chapter 2, not only are pesticides toxic at some level, they are increasingly ineffective. It now takes two to five applications of pesticide to accomplish what one application could do in the early

1970s. More than 500 insect pests, 270 weed species, and 150 plant diseases have developed resistance to one or more pesticides, making them harder to control[1] So to combat pests without as much dependence on pesticides, IPM uses complex controls ... lots of them. Biological, chemical, and cultural controls are the categories most often used to describe IPM practices. For example, instead of planning the date for using a fungicide on apples, pathologists monitor weather conditions with detail-driven equipment. This way they can tell if the disease that attacks during cold and wet springs has begun its ascent. If it has been hot and sunny, they can eliminate that day's chemical invasion — the chemical control. On the cultural control side, in the fall before the fated illness, growers would carefully remove from the ground any fallen apples or leaves that house the dreaded bacteria over the winter. And for a biological control, according to Tom Green of the IPM Institute of North America, "Growers might spray a nitrogen-rich urea treatment before leaf fall in autumn. The spray will cause the leaves to decompose more rapidly than untreated leaves through the action of microorganisms in the soil. Fewer leaves left intact in the spring translates into fewer viable apple scab spores to infect the new season's growth."[2]

> **"Being an IPM control freak in the field is certainly better than spraying all sorts of chemicals by the calendar."**

I watched the use of simple tools from the UMass apple IPM toolbox during the late spring of 1992 (before I knew I was pregnant). I had the fortunate opportunity to learn how to be a scout, a critical player in any IPM program. A scout is usually highly educated about a particular crop, the crop's beneficial and damaging insects, the environment of the region and acreage under examination, and the most up-to-date tools of pest management (at that point my training in the field was too short to call me highly educated!).

Traipsing about the apple orchards of Massachusetts with our leader, Margaret Christie, I examined the undersides of leaves and counted the marks left by a variety of insects. I learned about our most vicious disease, apple scab, which lies in wait over the winter in the "drops"(fallen apples) and leaves under the trees, and appears in the spring after a warm, wet spell. I saw the effects of voles on the rootstocks of young, newly planted trees, and the subsequent need for building small circular fences around the bases. Later in Ron Prokopy's lab (my new assignment with baby growing), I learned and counted the identifying marks of the insect plum curculio in apples and examined mites on leaves under a microscope. (One of my most exciting discoveries emerged under that lens ... read ahead.) In a very short time, I glimpsed the complexity of possibilities that exist in a creative IPM system.

War?

As I write these words describing our enemies – diseases, weeds, and insects – and the continuous battles we wage against them, I cannot help but find similarities to the war we may wage at any moment. Last night (September 28, 2001) I watched nine humongous military air carriers and three helicopters fly overhead within 90 minutes, all heading for Afghanistan.

I think of the enemies of our food that live among us, just as terrorists are reported to be. And I think of the arsenal we overuse to blast out the repugnant – the chemicals with which we ambush ourselves, causing cancer, polluted drinking water, and toxic fields, all in the name of protecting our food. Will our attempts to eradicate terrorism be as futile as our war against plant pests?

What have we learned from this centuries-long struggle? We have been met by new, resistant warriors – terrorists that emerge from hiding after mutating into superbugs, superweeds, superpathogens – that won't give up their commitment, as if the meaning of their lives is to annihilate green growth.

We have learned that direct combat is but a stopgap, with long-standing, irreversible damage as a result. We have learned that a sound alternative is a sustainable system, one that understands the enemy, that provides alternatives, focused not on weaponry but on healthy management practices. We have learned that we can be successful only by tracking populations, allowing leeway for sharing of the harvest, by letting Mother Nature instruct us on fair play.

We see a successful future that depends on a set of peace talks with those who can't talk. So we must behave and treat others, even our enemies, as we would want to be treated.

So what does IPM mean? I certainly don't want to venture into the definition debate this early on, so instead let's look at the practices it entails. I like to look at IPM as a toolbox of very complex and complicated, but relatively easy to apply, practices that consider all the elements of an agricultural ecosystem and only use chemicals as a last resort. Some people focus on the management of pests, while others focus on the management of the ecosystem. (More on the spectrum of application later.)

The production system is similar to that of organic practices in that the manager must understand the interaction of all the various components — agronomy, pathology, entomology, weed science, agricultural economics, etc. — to make integrated decisions. A systems-thinking approach really helps here. When I took the UMass IPM short course in January 1993, it was exactly three weeks before I delivered my first child, so my capacity for a complex systems approach was rather limited. I did understand pretty quickly, though, that it takes a variety of disciplines to fully comprehend IPM — the course was taught by a handful of professors and extension personnel from different departments. Thankfully, I had a baseline understanding of each of these areas and was actually thrilled to weave them together into practices that made sense.

> "I like to look at IPM as a toolbox of very complex and complicated, but relatively easy to apply, practices that consider all the elements of an agricultural ecosystem and only use chemicals as a last resort."

The first basic tenet of an IPM program is the monitoring of pests of all kinds, from insects to weeds. A scout usually does this with an economic threshold for the crop in mind, the second basic tenet of IPM. These thresholds consider potential injury levels and market value and are based on the pest's population, competition, behavior (will it be migrating or changing life cycle soon?), and environmental components. These thresholds usually take a lot of big-brain thinking. Biological, cultural, and chemical controls are the tools or the "many little hammers" (a simple but descriptive phrase coined by two weed ecologists)[3] used by farmers to practice IPM.

Like taking Echinacea when the first sign of a cold comes on, farmers apply IPM practices such as rotating crops, using disease-resistant plants, and irrigating early to help strengthen their crops for the season's onslaught. Sustainable agriculture consultant and advocate Chuck Benbrook says, "Promoting plant growth and strong defense mechanisms is clearly integral to sound pest management, just as good health and a sound immune system help people resist the flu and recover more quickly from health problems when they occur."[4]

Some of the practices scientists are coming up with are amazing. For example, in the early 1990s, biologists at Cornell University developed a potato variety with sticky leaf hairs that repelled beetles and aphids, while entomologists at Washington State University were experimenting with a common potato-field weed that beetles found so tasty they ignored nearby potatoes.[5]

With so little research on organics at universities, you might be surprised at how much is going on under the rubric of Integrated Pest Management. Since many of the solutions demand highly educated input, the land grant universities around the country have been contributing heavily to the basket of offerings. Some of these solutions are clearly applicable to organic production.

First, the bugs

The leaders of the IPM movement range from plant pathologists to entomologists. Although many of the solutions fall under other areas of study, damage we can relate to most readily seems to come from insects. First, let's look at the task given to bug scientists: can they, knowing all they do about life cycles, migration habits, culinary interests, and the like, come up with ever-changing battle plans? There is an enormous amount to understand about each insect and each crop, and all the multiples of that interaction. As entomologist Pamela Marrone puts it, "Instead of focusing on the pest in one field only, pest management includes knowledge on pest movement and migration patterns from location to location and pest behavior from one crop to another (e.g., understanding corn earworm/cotton bollworm ... as it moves from corn to cotton over a season; armyworm ... or Colorado potato beetle as it moves from overwintering sites at field edges into potato fields)."[6] I once took a graduate course in entomology, and I remember complaining to my husband that I felt as if I was in med school for bugs. In the lab final, we had to be able to locate the ovary of a grasshopper under a microscope — ugh!

Entomologists need to understand just about everything about pest behavior to develop their tactics. One of the most successful approaches is to use pheromones — the smell females give off when they are ready to mate— to confuse or attract the pest. An example of pheromone confusion is used at the Randall Island Project to reduce the use of Guthion, an organophosphate used to control "codling moth" in apples in that area. A tiny quantity of the attractant is placed on twist-ties that are then placed high up in trees. About 400 twist-ties per acre will fill an orchard with enough scent to thoroughly confuse the male moths. Most of them become exhausted chasing the pheromone and do not find the females.[7] The females' unfertilized eggs are the beginning of the end for that population. Of course, environmental conditions have to be just right for the tactic to be really successful.

Part of my Prokopy lab work was the preparation of hundreds of red sticky spheres. These spheres were devised to simply monitor apple maggot flies, a key summer pest. The red ball would attract certain pests and the insect would then get stuck on the sticky goop. At some point, Ron tested an attractant apple odor to further attract and "catch" the insects. More and more, scientists are developing alternative baits, such as pheromone contraptions.

Another tactic is serving "delicacies" … luring insects away from one dinner plate to another and reenacting a bit of "Arsenic and Old Lace." For example, in the summer of 1997, the USDA began testing this kind of "bait and kill" program on five sites, primarily in the US corn belt, to control corn rootworm. As reported in *Agricultural Research*, "Crop dusting planes sprayed a bait made from powdered wild buffalo gourd root laced with a tiny dose of carbaryl (commonly known as Sevin) insecticide — the equivalent of about an ounce per acre …. Its attraction is so strong that beetles stop dead in their tracks when they sense it and switch from eating plant leaves and other parts to eat mostly bait."[8] Although substantial reduction in insecticide use is projected over the long term, these methods seem to me to be in constant need of revision. That is the whole point, isn't it? Resistance to pesticides is one of our biggest problems, so using one successful program to solve our problems just doesn't work in the long run. It is a good example, though, of the kind of trickery scientists are adding to the arsenal in IPM toolboxes.

> "Entomologists have applied the principles of the food chain to pest management problems. As the movie *The Lion King* explained to our children, certain things eat other things that eat other things and so on. Predator bugs such as ladybugs, predator mites, and others help the farmer combat the target."

Moving from offering carrots to wielding sticks, entomologists have applied the principles of the food chain to pest management problems. As the movie *The Lion King* explained to our children, certain things eat other things that eat other things and so on. Predator bugs such as ladybugs, predator mites, and others help the farmer combat the target. Using predators is the most common "biological control" tool. When the tool was first applied to fields and orchards, prices were very high, as were the risks. Thankfully, these controls are coming down in price, as indicated in a report sponsored by the Consumers Union: "The price per 1,000 predacious mites has declined from about $20.00 in 1980 to between $4.50 for large volume orders and $6.00 for most retail customers in 1995. The price of green lacewings has dropped by half."[9] A number of years ago, our local strawberry grower purchased $500 worth of ladybird beetles (ladybugs) as an IPM method and, due to some weird weather condition that day, they promptly flew away. That was a lot of money for little, if any, reward. Today those beetles might cost closer to $50, a more reasonable amount to gamble.

Remember my reference to the exciting discovery under the microscope in Prokopy's lab? I found my first predator mite, an exciting moment. I remember looking at that jewel-shaped, golden mite for a long, long time before I had the courage to call Ron down from his office. Yes! That was the hero — that little speck of a golden gem would be the undoing of some hoodlum of the apple orchard. In that moment, I glimpsed the satisfaction entomologists must feel when they find opportunities to save a little part of the world.

Then, the disease

Diseases seem trickier. Comparing diseases to insects, Joyce Strand, coordinator of the University of California Statewide IPM program, said, "Diseases have been much more difficult. They respond to temperature and moisture. Now there are several weather stations on the market that can measure leaf wetness, so we are looking to refine our disease prediction models."[10]

Plant pathologists talk about a disease triangle (described in depth in Chapter 3), where three sides must be present for a disease to occur: favorable environment, susceptible plant, and virulent pathogen. Preventive controls can help with both the susceptible plant part and the presence of the pathogen, but the favorable environment is something that needs close monitoring. New computer prediction programs focus on the last piece — they can measure humidity and temperature and compare those factors to the plants' growth stage and then to the life cycles of the pathogens.

Interestingly, a handful of companies have become actively involved with promoting IPM practices with their growers, and one, Campbell Soup, has focused on the disease issue. (I never would have thought of Campbell Soup as being a particularly environmentally friendly company — you just never know.) Again from Chuck Benbrook: "Campbell Soup Company, a project collaborator in California, has made great strides in Mexico, California, and Ohio in applying disease forecasting models in tomato, potato, and other crops ... Campbell Soup records show that across this acreage (200,000 acres under contract to Campbell's), fungicide applications have been reduced over 50 percent — from around 10 applications per acre to about 4."[11]

Another company that has taken the lead in IPM is Gerber. In North Carolina and Michigan, Gerber has worked with apple growers to reduce dependence on organophosphates by using pheromone-based alternatives. As baby food manufacturers, they are particularly concerned about pesticides. Remember, when we see this kind of good behavior from big companies, we need to thank them and encourage them to stay the course as models to others.

And of course, the weeds

Finally there are the weeds. We learned in Chapter 2 about the dependence on herbicides in conventional agriculture. Weeds are tricky. An example of innovative mechanical practices for weed management is at Lange Twins Vineyard, one of the farms in the Lodi area, which comprises 16 percent of California's wine grape production. The famous wine region has been heralded in recent years for its commitment to constantly upgrading and improving its IPM practices. Lange Twins uses a variety of techniques, centering on native grass cover crops and composting, with the goal of creating healthy, balanced vineyards that can withstand disease and insect pressure. The vineyard does use Roundup in the vine rows at the rate of 1.5 pints per acre, down from the previous application of two quarts. It is applied from a machine pulled by a four-wheel motorcycle, which uses less water than a traditional applicator.[12]

The essence of IPM is the development of a complex and integrated plan. As Tom Green puts it, "IPM works best when growers, entomologists, plant pathologists, agronomists, weed scientists, economists, sociologists, etc., all work together on the production system as a whole to design an approach that is economically and environmentally sound, and within the means of the grower to adopt. Otherwise you end up with a basketful of different solutions, some of which might actually make other problems worse!"[13] Identifying how one solution could affect another and ensuring a balanced direction makes such sense —simple, but so difficult.

Along the spectrum

One of the most frustrating elements of IPM is that individual growers decide how much control to use. They may choose to hire a scout. They may use cover crops and build vegetative buffers around stream banks to minimize chemical runoff, but not reduce their use of certain pesticides. The interpretation of IPM varies widely from grower to grower and from scientist to scientist. I have spoken to university researchers who look at IPM as a way to help growers justify their sprays and others who look at IPM as a way to help growers off their pesticide addiction.

The intention of IPM is to reduce chemical use to zilch, unless serious pest out-breaks occur. Sadly, drug use on the fields has increased while we have worked so hard to "Just say no!" The General Accounting Office report on the implementation of IPM at the federal level clearly documents the sad state of our pesticide use. "IPM as implemented to this point has not yet yielded nationwide reductions in chemical pesticide use. In fact, total use of agricultural pesticides, measured in pounds of active ingredient, has actually increased since the beginning of USDA's IPM initiative."[14] The good news behind the bad is that use of the most toxic ver-sions is clearly dropping.

The report goes on to say that pesticide reduction was never the program's primary expectation. The actual intention of the federal program was quite different. In a backgrounder to the National IPM Initiative, we find these statistics: "On September 22, 1993, the Clinton administration, in joint testimony before Congress given by the leadership of USDA, USEPA, and FDA, stated that, 'implementing IPM practices on 75 percent of the nation's crop acres by the year 2000 was a national goal.'"[15] In actuality, at its lowest levels, the USDA came close. "USDA estimates that some level of IPM had been implemented on about 70 percent of the nation's crop acreage as of the end of crop year 2000, only slightly short of USDA's 75-percent goal."

At the time the program was first announced, the USDA was not sure how many acres were under IPM production. It came out that somewhere around 50 percent of the total US acreage could be counted as using IPM. That was a big part of the problem: "counted." The system tabulated use of a scout, economic thresholds, and then whether or not a farmer used one, two, or three different IPM-like practices.

It is hardly a surprise that the government system was based on quantity of practices ("indicative of an IPM approach") without much complexity. It certainly would be easier to manage the paperwork. With such variability in the criteria, growers would have less difficulty reaching the requirement, and everyone could go home without an argument ... and without much change. In the end, growers could count practices that were not even intended to reduce pesticides. The GAO report noted that "crop acreage can be counted in the IPM estimate even if growers use a combination of practices that may result in little or no reduction in pesticide use."[16]

So then some do-gooders came along and demanded tighter standards. They wanted more prevention plus less toxicity and more selectivity of the pesticides that *are* used. They wanted change. Thank goodness.

Biointensive IPM

Chuck Benbrook and his demands for higher levels of IPM are well known. The Protected Harvest label, currently on Wisconsin-grown potatoes and presumably other fruits and vegetables in the future, verifies the use of biointensive standards.

"Biointensive IPM is a systems approach to pest management that is based on an understanding of pest ecology. It relies on resistant varieties and promoting plant health, crop rotation, disrupting pest reproduction, and the management of biological processes to diversify and build populations of beneficial organisms. Reduced-risk pesticides, including biopesticides, are used only as a last resort and only in ways that minimize risks."

One of them was Chuck Benbrook, who was working with the Consumers Union to demand greater accountability and stricter definitions around IPM. His report, "Pest Management at the Crossroads," became an important document for change in the industry. Referring to a June 1996 *California Farmer* article describing a "strict" IPM program for cotton insect pest management, Chuck said, "If a spray program including four different chemical families and six to eight applications can be called 'strict IPM,' especially in California, a new definition of IPM is needed." He continued, "Unfortunately, the USDA's definition of IPM and its adoption criteria were quite lax, and we believe the Economic Research Service analysis overstates actual progress along the continuum by a wide margin."[17]

Even though the intention of Vernon Stern (who, with his co-workers at the University of California, first started IPM in 1959) was to focus on an ecological balance, the biology of the system became secondary to "scout and spray" application. The farmer calculated an economically tolerable level of pest populations, hired scouts to determine if pests had surpassed this level, and sprayed if they had.[18] Chuck has fought for more biologically based practices in his biointensive IPM definition. The General Accounting Office reported that, while the USDA estimated that IPM was implemented on 76 percent of corn acreage in 2000, biologically-based IPM practices were implemented on no more than 18 percent of corn acreage.[19]

The USDA did try to define the practices in a way they could tabulate, to encourage further improvements. By 1997, it had a new definition that focused on a

Levels of IPM

Tom Green of the IPM Institute of North America wrote the standards for the Food Alliance, probably the first national IPM label we will see. Tom's system awards points, depending on the level of IPM implemented.

Level 1: No IPM

Inputs are applied on a preventive basis, without systematic monitoring, testing, or sampling to determine actual need or best timing. Level One practices represent the minimum qualification for grower participation, e.g., minimum legal requirements for pesticide application records. If any Level One practice is applicable and not met, the participant is immediately disqualified.

Level 2: Low Level IPM

Inputs are applied according to need, as determined by monitoring, testing, or sampling. Low Level IPM is characterized by the following general practices:

- weather-monitoring/forecasting systems are employed to determine the best timing for input application;
- computer software is used to interpret scouting or forecasting system data;
- sampling routines are used to collect information on pest levels, crop phenology, and nutrition status;
- pest-monitoring traps, sweep nets, and magnifiers are used to sample pests;
- a professional crop consultant, scout, or trained in-house scout is employed to perform sampling routines;
- pest-resistance strategies are employed;
- thresholds are used to make decisions on input use.

Level 3: Medium Level IPM

Efforts are made to reduce the use of high-risk and broad-spectrum pesticides, to protect beneficial organisms and farm workers.

- available pesticides are ranked by risk level, and those with the least risk are employed whenever possible;
- cultural pest-control measures are used to reduce use and doses of chemical pesticides;
- pest habitats are modified or removed to improve biodiversity;
- alternate-row spraying is used to create refuges for beneficials and to reduce amounts of pesticides applied.

Level 4: High Level IPM

Preventive measures are employed to reduce the need for in-season intervention.

- pest-resistant crop varieties are planted;
- crop rotations are used specifically to reduce input needs;
- crops are selected that require the least amount of intervention in-season;
- advanced and at times more expensive pest-management options are selected, including mating disruption and biopesticides, and applied when thresholds indicate need;
- natural enemies are augmented with applications of beneficial organisms;
- soil quality is monitored and improved.

management strategy for prevention, avoidance, monitoring, and suppression of pest populations, the PAMS approach. To be considered IPM, tactics had to be in use from three or more of these components.

IPM definitions were being batted about; for example, ecological pest management was introduced as an alternative. A continuum concept seemed the most consistent compromise for the industry. Steve Balling, an IPM specialist with Del Monte Foods, introduced this concept around 1994, the continuum running from conventional, chemical-based pest management systems to "systems pest management" reliant on information and biological controls.[20] Many others have adopted the idea of levels of IPM and have included it in their own standard setting.

I feel about IPM as I do about organics. The jury may still be out, but while we aren't sure, I

Shopping tip

"Protected Harvest standards fall on the end I want to be on: bio-intensive IPM."

will stick with looking closely at the standards and seeing where they sit on the continuum. I know, for example, that Protected Harvest standards fall on the end I want to be on: biointensive IPM.

So if pesticides are not to be used except as a true last resort, what is the difference between an organic system and a well-handled IPM system? Some say organic growers can actually use more toxic compounds, albeit natural, such as pyrethrumone and other heavy-duty sprays, than a dedicated IPM grower might. When I asked Tom Green of the IPM Institute of North America to answer that very needling question, he replied, "I envision bio-intensive IPM and high-level organic as close to an intersection of the two systems, where you've designed the system from the start to be self-sustaining without intervention — choosing the crops, the varieties, planting systems to match the site-specific environment; prepared the soil and adjacent non-cropping areas to maximize plant health, etc. Then you can sit back and watch the season unfold with minimal intervention. IPM growers have a broader range of intervention options when needed than do organic growers, but other than that, there's very little difference at the high end of the continuum of both systems."

Weigh the ways ... local and IPM may top your priority list

Here's the tricky part. If you prize locally-grown and your farmer uses high-level IPM practices in every way, it should be your product of choice. Growers using IPM practices face barriers everyday. IPM information comes from sources that they rarely see anymore — certainly not their regular chemical salespeople. New IPM management practices are often odd-sounding and are in the very experimental stages when growers are asked to try them. And technically, IPM management is complicated and taxing, and ultimately may be more expensive for farmers. With all this in mind, our role becomes ever more important. Supporting IPM practices with our purchases is the most immediate way of endorsing their efforts and encouraging them to stay with it for yet another day. It's up to us ... every day, choosing supper in a way that is good for you and good for the Earth.

> "Supporting IPM practices with our purchases is the most immediate way of endorsing their efforts and encouraging them to stay with it for yet another day."

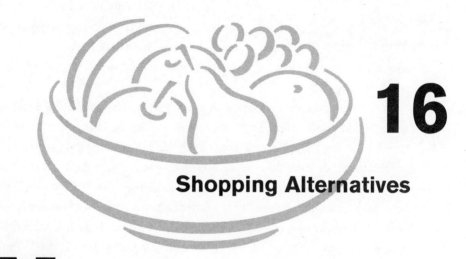

16

Shopping Alternatives

MOST OF US GO TO THE GROCERY STORE 2.7 TIMES PER WEEK. How do we find our eco-foods, and what can we do to encourage more options for our eco-bellies? There are a few tricks to keep in mind while shopping for environmentally sound foods. Some of these we can do at our local grocery. Other options we certainly want to consider are shopping at more earth-friendly retailers, farmers' markets, and roadside stands. Let's start where we find ourselves the most often.

Going to the grocery store

Most of us don't need to look at the current market research, which says we just don't like grocery shopping. "Get in and get out!" That's my motto. It's hard to believe we go as often as we do. Once a month might be more efficient, but it just doesn't work that way. I am always trying to stretch one week's shopping into two. Animal and fish protein for the first week, lentils, pasta, and soups served up the second. It takes a bit of time to plan, and who's got that anymore? So how do we grocery shop and spend the extra time to find the eco-foods we need?

Most grocers send out circulars each week with highlighted and sale products. Throw them out! By the time this book gets into your hands, things may have changed, but today, circulars just don't highlight much in the way of natural

> ## Shopping tip
> *"Always check the place of origin, and buy local if you can."*

products or organic produce. Planning the week's purchases with circulars might have worked in the past, but unless you have a good eco-discipline, on-sale items of not-all-that-good-for-you stuff can be alluring. They certainly pull me in. I love to save money, but circulars do not tell you the stories you now know. So unless your store features its on-sale organics, recycle the circular!

In Chapter 1, we took a tour down the aisles. Now let's summarize a few key things to help ease the effort. First, zip by the on-sale items. I scan with my eyes and keep the cart moving just in case. I have a very hard time letting go of sale items.

Next, little labels dot the produce, and grocery signs tell us more. What to look for? Always check the place of origin, and buy local if you can. (Part of the current Farm Bill is an amendment seeking to assure produce is labeled with place of origin. Let's hope it passes — we need to know!) Second, production method ... check for organic, IPM, low spray, or Demeter/Biodynamic (wouldn't that be nice?). Third,

> ## Shopping tip
> *"Production method ... check for organic, IPM, low spray, or Demeter/Biodynamic."*

producer ... is it a big agribusiness, a small farm, or a farmers' cooperative? If you get too frustrated with the lack of information, ask your produce manager. With more people asking questions, they are bound to get the hint. "We need to know!"

On to the processed foods ... there is clearly much more to read in these aisles. Yes, this takes a bit more energy, but remember, the research doesn't have to happen at every visit. Find your favorites and double-check periodically for new products. The number of new natural products far outpaces regular products, but the natural ones still don't hit the shelves as often as

> ## Shopping tip
> *"Producer... is it a big agri-business, a small farm, or a farmers' cooperative?"*

we might think. If you have a special natural or organic section, head there first while you have some energy. As my children remind me, they love the natural section — they can usually con Mom into buying many more treats there.

In the meat section look for antibiotic-free, free-range, free-farmed, or organic eco-labels, or any other wording referring to humane treatment. Be wary of the word "natural" — you will find it overused by companies of questionable repute. In the fish section, take one of the handy cards referred to in Chapter 12, unless you have favorites you have already researched and approved. In the dairy section, look for rBGH- or rBST-free, organic and/or local. If local is your favorite, you might want to call the dairy and ask about hormone additives. Remember that humane treatment of dairy cows is also a good thing. Keep an eye out for any reference to it on their packages.

> **Shopping tip**
>
> *"In the meat section look for antibiotic-free, free-range, free farmed, or organic eco-labels, or any other wording referring to humane treatment."*

Throughout the store, remember to look for eco-labels, such as Protected Harvest, the Food Alliance, Marine Stewardship Council, and Fair Trade Coffee. If you see a label you are unsure of, but like the way it looks, check **<www.eco-labels.org>** when you get home.

Once you are home, the real Sherlock Holmes work begins. To find the true clues, go to the Internet. Although a web presence is still fairly rare for small growers, most companies have websites. Go online and check their sites. What do they say about their practices? If they contribute a percentage of sales to a cause, find out more about it. Many websites have instant e-mail. Ask your questions. If you feel funny about asking, remember how many of your hard-earned dollars will go to that farmer. Your efforts matter!

> **Shopping tip**
>
> *"In the dairy section, look for rBGH- or rBST-free, organic and/or local."*

Where else can we go?

Been there, done that. Tired of going to the big old grocery store, trying to find a needle in a haystack? You may find relief at one of the natural foods grocery stores — Whole Foods, Trader Joe's, etc. — or a smaller independent grocer who emphasizes natural foods. Don't forget the folks who helped kickstart the movement, the "health food" stores.

Natural grocers have mushroomed in recent years; Canada is just being served up a slew of these stores. We have also seen their numbers grow in the US. Whole Foods, for example, owns approximately 120 stores in the US, with

> **Shopping tip**
>
> *"Throughout the store, remember to look for eco-labels, such as Protected Harvest, the Food Alliance, Marine Stewardship Council, and Fair Trade Coffee."*

approximately 20,000 products in each. In the past few years, the natural products industry has been concerned that consumers would reduce their trips to these stores as conventional grocers add new items. So far, that has not happened. A recent article in *Natural Foods Merchandiser*, one of the industry's trade publications, reported that "Natural products retailers are holding their market share against the long-predicted onslaught of the mass market, and still represent the largest portion of sales when functional foods [foods with specific health benefits] are excluded."[1]

Our local Whole Foods supermarket is Bread & Circus. B&C is always brimming with activity. Many of these stores have figured out how much we like an "experience" while shopping and have set up their stores to fulfill that desire. The other night, my husband and I stopped in to grab something before a movie and ended up having dinner there. It had been a while since we had stopped by, and we were both surprised by how much the dining area had expanded and how prepared-by-the-store foods had taken over the deli section.

I must reveal my secret. I have often perused the deli area with the notion of replicating the dish at home. Many of these delicacies, in their ready-to-go form, are beyond my budget. Not to be deterred, I look closely at the list of ingredients, go back to the aisles for the products and keep my fingers crossed in the kitchen at home. I am afraid I must also reveal that the deli's successes far outpace my own.

One of the nicest things about these stores is that their staff is ready and willing to chat. They expect a lot of questions from a discerning buyer and usually know where things are from and how they were raised, a welcome treat. Their labeling is usually pretty good, too, although I find private labels (the stores' own name and logo) frustrating, as they leave me without much information. Otherwise, the stores do tend to provide more information, such as leaflets and signs, than the conventional stores. Our B&C has worked with CISA (Community Involved in Sustaining Agriculture), the local sustainable agriculture support and promotion group, to highlight farmers' faces and put their stories on signs throughout the stores. With those signs next to their products, you can make the connection a little more easily. The Food Alliance similarly provides stores in the Northwest with point-of-purchase materials. It is a wonderful service to shoppers!

To market, to market

Farmers' markets are a great way to get the food facts. Face to face with your farmer, here is a golden opportunity to find out how he grows, what his values are, and if his methods are something you want to support. Farmers' markets are also wonderful places to find fresh and nutritious products, knowing your money goes directly to the farm. Our farmers' market runs every Saturday morning and has become a bit of a social event for the community. You are pretty sure to see at least some of your neighbors. Markets vary around the country. Some are strictly for vegetables; others (like ours) expand to include cheeses, breads, herbs, and plants.

It must be noted that some farmers' markets around the country are hardly markets for farmers, allowing vendors of all kinds, including some who may buy vegetables from down the road and resell them to you at a higher price. There are even some who import fruits and vegetables from all over the globe and try to suggest they are local. Be careful! With this possibility in mind, you understand the importance of asking the tough questions — finding out who the farmers are and asking about their practices. In our market, farmers are not all organic or IPM or necessarily all reputable, so I ask.

> ## Shopping tip
>
> *"Farmers' markets are also wonderful places to find fresh and nutritious products, knowing your money goes directly to the farm."*

Sometimes, state or local organizations will help guarantee farmers' authenticity. In California, there over 350 communities with "certified" farmers' markets. In New York City, Greenmarket, the group that organizes and manages 28 farmers' markets for 175 farmers, has specific rules. Only regional growers are allowed to sell at the markets, and Greenmarket staff makes routine inspections.

In a small town in France while on a sustainable agriculture tour, I was treated to an organic-only farmers' market. Much smaller than the regular market, it was comforting to know ahead of time that all the growers there practiced the agriculture you wanted for your foodstuffs. No questions necessary. While we wait for the North American counterpart, we still need to ask the questions.

How to ask those tough questions of a farmer? It helps if he or she seems nice, but it really gets down to whether you are content with their practices. If you're anything like normal, you probably lose all your questions, just like in the doctor's office, the minute you see the expert. But, as in any new relationship, finding out what's there before jumping in is a good idea. The farmer wants you as a customer forever, so, as in a good dating service, getting the facts out of the way is a good place to start. I always begin with one or two simple questions attached to a compliment, like "These are beautiful greens. They must be organic ... right? " or "These apples look so crisp. Do you use IPM in your orchard?" That usually gets the ball rolling. If the grower looks at me funny on those two questions, I mosey on. If a farmer simply answers "yes," without getting excited enough to tell me more, I wonder, but wait until the next week to make a judgment call. He might simply have other things on his mind.

One of the highlights of a farmers' market is learning about value-added items. Today, many growers bring on-farm processed items along with their load of fresh ones. Herb growers bring tinctures and salves, grain growers bring breads, and flower growers bring dried arrangements. How they made these products is always interesting. Knowing that purchasing them further supports your neighbor and not an oversized corporate agribusiness is even better.

Farmers' markets have become a mainstay of the North American food shopping experience. According to the USDA, there are 19,000 farmers selling their produce at 2,800 farmers' markets in the US, the number having increased 63 percent from 1994 to 2000.[2] The USDA programs now include a WIC (Women, Infants, and Children) Farmers' Market Nutrition Program that provides coupons to WIC participants for purchasing fresh fruits and vegetables at many of the markets. This year, 58 percent of the farmers' markets participated. A similar program is just beginning for low-income senior citizens.

The USDA also maintains a list of local markets at **<www.ams.usda.gov/ farmersmarkets/map.htm>**. Sometimes a state's department of food and agriculture maintains the data. Either way, you don't need to miss a week, even when on vacation. Call ahead for farmers' market information in the area you are visiting, and you can have fresh food at the campsite.

In Canada, Toronto has a number of wonderful markets, and Farmers' Market Ontario maintains information and assistance for approximately 150 markets, reporting annual sales exceeding $500 million.[3]

Drive-through corn, lettuce, tomatoes, and more

A quick stop on the way home or a scenic drive can put you at roadside with some of the freshest local fare. From building a relationship with a local grower to developing your seasonal eating, watching the seasons pass at a roadside stand is a wonderful way to connect to the Earth's fruits.

No one seems to be able to count them, but there are plenty of roadside stands. Some stay open a season, others operate from late winter to early winter. You may already have your favorites lined up to and from work, or you may need to take a round trip to search them out. If you live in a city, a trip to the country may not take as long as you think. Some stands perch right outside city limits. Saturday morning seems to be a good time for finding stands, and sometimes even catching the farmer.

One of the best parts of roadside stands is the support for eating seasonally. Watching what is being served up each week (or month) gives us a true perspective on the seasonal cycle. When apples are ready, it's time for pies, applesauce, baked apples, apple crisp, and preserving dried apple rings. Another highlight is learning about different varieties and what they are best suited for. Depending on the number of roadside stands near you, you might find some are better than others for certain things. At one, the best sweet corn is Butter and Sugar, at another, the best sweet corn is Silver Queen. So much to try ... so much fun!

> "From building a relationship with a local grower to developing your seasonal eating, watching the seasons pass at a roadside stand is a wonderful way to connect to the Earth's fruits."

Pick-your-own and thank you

A group outing to a pick-your-own fall apple orchard or a spring strawberry field can guarantee fun for the gang and a real aid for your farmer. Labor is one of the most costly parts of farming. If you can lend a hand on that end, it can help. On the other hand, visiting pickers may not be helpful. Many growers who have attempted pick-your-own operations find it frustrating to watch nurtured plants trampled by the end of a day. Or when more apples are found on the ground than sold, farmers wonder if it is worth the assistance. So we have a part to play. Honoring their efforts and livelihood is our part. Providing good, ripe fruits or vegetables is theirs.

Pick-your-own operations are a bit easier to find than roadside stands, with the help of your state department of food and agriculture or on farm maps produced by local farming organizations. Some states have websites with maps, so it may be worth a visit to the Internet. Once you've found a nearby pick-your-own, call ahead to check picking conditions. The farm can tell you if the produce is ripe enough for good picking. Check on their hours and ask if you need to bring anything and if they have any policies you should know about ahead of time. Of course, by now, asking about their production practices is probably second nature.

As with roadside stands, there are some priceless aspects to the pick-your-own experience. Getting that close to the source of your food creates an appreciation you might never have experienced otherwise. Most exciting for a family, particularly with small children, are the glowing faces that naturally occur when picking fruit from the source. Children learn firsthand where their food comes from and how important the soil is. And if you have started to find the joys of putting up your own produce for later in the year, filling a basket with what will become a holiday treat is a very satisfying reward. Some operations offer value-added products, such as pies and turnovers. Remember, if you support the farm, buying extras helps tell the farmers you appreciate their efforts.

Farms are all different. Many have tempting side attractions, such as hayrides and petting zoos, to round out your on-farm experience. One farm not too far from here has campsites. Some have mailing lists to keep you up-to-date on their activities. One farm I know sends out postcards when the blueberries are ready for picking. Some farms have websites. You can map out a full day's tour of pick-your-own farms, and then settle in at one with a campsite.

17

If You Can't Beat 'em, Join 'em

JOIN THE FARM THAT IS ... the Community Supported (or Shared) Agriculture (CSA) movement is bringing us onto the farms, even if we live in cities. It's about foods as fresh as the dirt it grows in and as close to the source as anyone can get. One of the most exciting movements of our time, Community Supported Agriculture, exemplifies the alternative for which we have been searching. These farms are spreading like wildfire across the country. The system works for farmer and eater alike. Members pay an annual fee to share in the harvest, picking up their produce once a week. For the farmer, there's no need to find a market, because the market is the membership. Eaters get the chance to share in the harvest as well as in the risk. If corn borer ruins a crop, members feel the results. Most of the time, it's fresh, clean, good-for-the-soul food picked right from the soil. With family and friends around you, picking peas and squishing raspberries in your mouth constitutes the true spirit of community.

How it started

In the mid-1960s, a group of Japanese women concerned about maintaining the local flavor and economy of their foodstuffs developed a direct-buying relationship with some local farms and dubbed it "teikei" or "putting the farmers' face on food."

It started with 200 women buying milk direct. (Today it serves 230,000 households under the consumer alliance, the Seikatsu Club.)

This concept subsequently emerged in various parts of Europe and traveled overseas to New England in the mid-1980s. Two farms were simultaneously testing a variation of the concept in 1986, Temple-Wilton Community Farm in New Hampshire and Indian Line Farm in Massachusetts. The next year, our CSA, Brookfield Farm, jumped on the bandwagon along with several others, and the movement was off to the races.

Two advocates grew out of those first two farms, Trauger Groh in New Hampshire (who then assisted Brookfield and remained on our board for many years) and Robyn VanEn in Massachusetts. Trauger Groh wrote books and papers on the emerging model, with much emphasis on biodynamic farming, and Robyn VanEn became the voice for adoption of CSA.

The CSA movement emanates from the resource center named in her honor: the Robyn VanEn Center housed at Wilson College in Pennsylvania. She became known as the foremost pioneer of the movement as she shared the concept with pride and passion throughout the country as speaker, organizer, educator, and advocate. She also traveled to Russia to share alternatives with farmers there. She was the founder of CSA of North America and was well-known for her tireless efforts in building a foundation for CSA. Her untimely death in 1997 was a shock to many in the movement. Her work will long be remembered.

Today there are approximately 1,000 CSA farms (that's a pretty rapid increase in just 15 years) throughout North America, mostly in the Northeast, along with groups in Minnesota, Wisconsin, and California's Bay Area.[1] At the third Northeast Community Supported Agriculture Conference, while a majority of participants came from the Northeast, many came from places such as California, Louisiana, Kentucky, North Carolina, Michigan, Ontario, Quebec, New Mexico, Arizona, Texas, Oregon, and even Australia and Azerbaijan. (CSAs are also cropping up in places like Atlanta and Kalamazoo.)

According to research administered by the Northeast Sustainable Agriculture Working Group (NESAWG) with a grant from the Northeast Sustainable Agriculture Research and Education Program (NESARE) of the United States Department of Agriculture (USDA) (there will be an acronym quiz at the end of this chapter), nearly 95 percent of CSA farmers use organic or biodynamic practices. VanEn said, "The main goal of these community-supported projects is to develop participating farms to their highest ecological potential and to develop a network that will encourage and allow other farms to become involved."[2] After witnessing the 350-plus participants at a recent CSA conference share their enthusiasm for ecological and community-based operations, I would say that goal is well on its way to being reached.

CSA is a model that excites the palate and the soul. As an eater, you enjoy the best food there is; as a citizen, you know you are doing "the right thing" by contributing to a food system of recovery. It quietly and gently wins the argument for a just and sustainable food system by just doing it — offering ecologically sound farming practices in relation with a community that cares.

> "CSA is a model that excites the palate and the soul. As an eater, you enjoy the best food there is; as a citizen, you know you are doing "the right thing" by contributing to a food system of recovery"

How it works

Joining a farm doesn't mean you'll pick up a hoe or sit behind the wheel of one of those really cool-looking tractors, although you may be asked to contribute some elbow grease along the way. It means that you pay a certain fee for the season, based on all the expenses of running the farm, divided by the number of members. It may mean you show up once a week for "pickup," getting your share of the harvest. Depending on where you live and how your CSA farm operates, you may be asked to pick your own week's worth of some crops, such as beans, herbs, and raspberries. Some farms have monthly parties, others simply hold an annual meeting once a year. The season of your harvest also depends on where you live, how your CSA operates, and where it is located. In some areas the season may run from early June to Thanksgiving; in others, almost the whole year. However it's run, there is no better way to experience the fortune of life around farming.

With sturdy blinders in place, I thought for a long time that the Brookfield Farm model was the norm, and even though I was a speaker at the first CSA conference years ago, I must not have heard others around me. Then again, in very short order, new, creative types are joining the movement and expanding it in unique ways. But there are some core components for most farms — let's walk through a typical experience from the Brookfield vantage point and share, here and there, different approaches at other farms.

For most prospective CSA members, the experience begins through word of mouth. It might go something like this: The mom of one of your daughter's friends in preschool is waiting with you while the girls yell, "Just five more minutes, pleeeease!" She checks her watch and says, "We've got to stop at the farm before supper." You say, "What farm?" She says, "Oh, we belong to Brookfield Farm. We pick up fresh produce once a week, and this week the peas and strawberries are in, so we'll do some picking." You say, "You mean you go out to the field and pick fresh fruits and vegetables?" She says, "Yes — sometimes it's a little embarrassing — I can't get little Suzy here to stop stuffing herself full. By the time we get home, she has eaten so many, she hardly wants to eat dinner." You think, "This woman is complaining about her daughter eating too many fresh fruits and vegetables?! I'm lucky to get anything healthy into my children!" However, out loud you say, "So, how does one join the farm? Can I start right away?"

Then you call the farm and ask the details. It either sends you a brochure or directs you to its website, because farmers are always on the move. What you find out from this information is the cost of the "share." That is what you are buying, after all: a share of the harvest. (Brookfield produces 5–18 pounds of produce per member per week, depending on the time of year.) If Mother Nature gives you a smooth season, you will have lots of yummy goodies to share with the membership. If it is rather bumpy (too little/too much rain, too many insects, etc.), you will have fewer of those goodies to share. You will, however, understand a little bit more about the reality of what it takes to get food from field to plate.

You will be lucky if you have savvy, friendly farmers. For example, at Brookfield last year, we had a squash problem. (I think it had to do with a frost pocket we are in.) The farm down the road, the Food Bank Farm, had a great squash year, but got clobbered by hail and ran low on something else, of which we had plenty. Thankfully, we don't have a competitive relationship. To the contrary, our Farmer Dan and theirs, Michael Doctor, seem to be good buds — enough to do the old switcheroo and make everyone at both farms very happy.

Back to the cost of the share … according to the CSA census referenced earlier, the average cost of a share is $410, half-shares at $263. Remember, that is the price for many, many weeks of fresh produce and, potentially, other items. Most farms have conducted a price analysis and have determined the price ends up somewhere between organic and conventional prices in the grocery store. How much produce or other items, such as herbs, fruits, flowers, etc., are in a share versus a half-share depends on the farm. In Brookfield's case, we have one share size, with two payment types: $325 per share if you pay in January, and $350 if you need to pay over time. This encourages early paying, which helps the cash flow, an extremely important support for the farm budget. This was one of the benefits of the original CSA model: paying before the season begins funds the process when it is needed most.

For those farms that offer either a share or half-share (Brookfield used to offer both, so I remember the difficulty of decision-making), it may be a tough choice the first year. Depending on your family size, if you know you want to put food up, then throw caution to the wind and try the full share. If you are in the testing-the-waters stage, take a half-share and finish the season wanting more. I always felt a full share was too much (when we had the option), and yet I envied those who took the full load. I knew they were happy, healthy families eating loads of locally grown, put-up veggies in the dead of winter. Even last night, as I ate frozen peas from a bag, I bemoaned my lack of effort this past June. What a difference it makes to look at a fully stocked freezer or tomato jars lining our kitchen counter throughout the snowy months.

What do you get in your share? That will depend on the size of your farm and the ingenuity of your farmer. Five Springs Farm in northwestern Michigan runs a 20-week CSA for 36 shares on one-and-a-half acres of raised beds, and yet they still provide an interesting, marvelous array of goodies. "In April we harvest over-wintered leeks, parsnips, and Jerusalem artichokes, often dug up in the snow. These early vegetables are a real treat for our winter-weary members. We grow over 30 different veggies; lettuce and spring mix are our specialties. Most weeks our shareholders get a bouquet and herbs."[3] All on one-and-a-half acres of raised beds!

Some farms have different types of shares that can be added to the main share. For example, Silver Creek Farm in Ohio has meat shares, with lamb, beef, and chicken. It also offers goat milk cheese, a knitting share (for sweaters and mittens knit from fiber produced on the farm), and sometimes even a beer share with members brewing beer and dividing the bottled product at the end.[4]

You will also learn from a farm's brochure how long the season runs. Some farms run special "winter" shares or other shortened versions; some lucky ones in warmer climates run a longer season. For the most part, seasons run from May or June until October or November. Brookfield starts the first weekend in June, with final pickup the Tuesday before Thanksgiving. It is always a bittersweet day for me. Collecting all those butternut squash, potatoes, kale, onions, Brussels sprouts, pumpkins for pie, celeriac, and the turkey itself (since Dan works with a local poultry farmer to bring us fresh birds) is very exciting, knowing the feast will be made from fresh, local, organic food. It is also one of the saddest days

> "Collecting all those butternut squash, potatoes, kale, onions, Brussels sprouts, pumpkins for pie, celeriac, and the turkey itself is very exciting, knowing the feast will be made from fresh, local, organic food."

197

Kale

It's kale season! At our farm, that starts around July and continues through Thanksgiving. When we first became members of Brookfield, I wondered about the enormous crinkly leaves that seemed to wait patiently for my reach. A little leathery and worn, yet deep green and robust, the leaves quietly boasted of more nutrition then I could have guessed.

Kale is packed with calcium, 90 mg per serving, and recommended by the American Dietetic Association, especially for women. I fit the profile for osteoporosis: woman, thin, fair, blonde, and I need all the calcium I can get, especially when sardines with bones is an alternative source.

So I finally gave into kale's stoic stare, thanks to a dinner party where it was well prepared. Now it's all the rage in our family. How can seven- and eight-year-olds find happiness in kale? Go figure. A little steaming, a little olive oil and garlic help. Maybe they intuitively know they need it. For whatever reason, it works. You'll find kale in season at the Barstows in soup, sautéed, steamed with lemon and pepper, or mixed with other greens and tomatoes over pasta. Here is one of my favorites:

Portuguese (or some kind of adaptation of) Kale Soup

- 1 smoked sausage, kielbasa or (to be authentic) Choricio (hot Portuguese sausage), or anything you can get locally or antibiotic-free, sliced $1/2$" thick
- 1 tablespoon olive oil
- 1 quart free-range antibiotic-free chicken broth
- 1 medium onion, thinly sliced
- 3 medium potatoes, cubed
- 1 large bunch kale, shredded

Place olive oil and onions in a large pot to sauté slightly. Add washed sausage and sauté enough to render the fat; remove some of the grease with a paper towel. Add chicken broth, potatoes, and kale and cook for fifteen minutes or so.

of the year, knowing I will soon be heading to the grocery store again. I will miss the apprentices, chatting with other members, the children begging for homemade frozen yogurt pops made with fresh berries. But the good news is that if the season is bountiful, as it was this past year, I will be welcome in the cooler and greenhouses to pick up squash, sweet potatoes, pumpkins, carrots, rutabagas, collard greens, daikon radishes, parsnips, and drying red chili peppers as long as they last. What a treat! Not all farms run this way. Most of the farms that provide this fare do so under a winter share agreement — root crops for another couple of months at another price.

When and where do you pick up your weekly gold mine? That depends on where your farm is and who does the distributing. In our case, we are very lucky to have three "Farm Shop" days to choose from: Saturday mornings from 8:00 a.m. to 1:00 p.m. and Tuesday and Thursday afternoons from 3:00 p.m. to 7:00 p.m. When the kids get off the school bus, we go directly to the farm and pick up our share. In addition to our Amherst members, we have 150 members in Boston who receive their shares at one of three different locations in the Boston area once a week. They don't receive the pick-your-own produce in lieu of delivery. On the other hand, Farmer Dan has always encouraged Boston members to come out to the farm to pick whenever they want. I have been at the farm when these city dwellers come out and do the deep-inhaling routine. They can't seem to get enough of the farm smell — all the flowers, the herbs, the berries, the soil. Even one frozen Thanksgiving weekend, a Boston member who arrived to share in the extra bounty of the cooler seemed to be deep-breathing, and there weren't too many smells happening at that point. There is just something about being at the farm. It "feels right."

> **"There is just something about being at the farm. It "feels right.""**

Many farms around the country deliver to urban areas. In some cases, the membership delivers. One core shareholder will pick up and bring the goodies back to the neighborhood, to be picked up from someone's front porch, a church, or other community locale. Members may never see the farm except on an occasional "work day" or just for a visit. Thankfully, the goodness of the farm speaks through every mouthful of harvest. The main role of a member is to eat and appreciate.

Even a choice of three pickups can be difficult for this overly-committed working mom. It helps me out a lot that the pick-your-own items can be picked whenever it's convenient. When the children and I have an hour before some event, we stop at the farm to get that week's cherry tomatoes and green beans. Needless to say, they may never make it back for a meal. Snack time is transformed — out go the pretzels, in come the tomatoes and beans. I love that farm!

So, new member, you know when to come, how much you'll get, and what it costs — so let's go! You arrive at the farm on the first day to be greeted by the fashionably tan apprentices. (How did they get that color? Work the fields from 6 a.m. to 6 p.m. every day, and you can sport a tan in early June, too). They will show you the "boards." Two of the boards will list the "share" for that day. Brookfield Farm works on a mix-and-match system, but many farms simply tell you what to take, meaning one of this, a pound of that, etc. Brookfield tells individuals what size bag to use and lets them decide what goes in it. I have been known to fill a bag with spinach instead of small quantities of all the greens, particularly when I am having a party or putting something up for the winter. It has not always been this way. For years we picked up our share by the item. Although we ended up with a few more radishes than we wanted, it stretched our palates and made me get more creative with menu planning. For that, I will be forever grateful.

In addition to the share boards at Brookfield, there is a pick-your-own board, which lists what is ready in the fields and how much to pick of each item. There is always something on the board. In the height of the summer, a bouquet of flowers is part of the share. Having a beautiful bouquet of flowers in the middle of the table all summer feels luxurious and grand. Even after frost, herbs are available, some of which have become significant crops. For example, Dan grows basil successively throughout the season so people can put up pesto whenever they like. Other favored herbs are cilantro, parsley, and dill, as well as chives, sage, oregano, and the rest of the usual culinary herbs.

The final board describes the activities at the farm, perhaps a celebration coming up or a meat-sale day. Brookfield is a biodynamic farm, and its farm animals make it a fully integrated system. Periodically, the farm will make beef or pork products available for sale. At one time, the farm considered a chicken share, which would have allowed individuals to sign up for a chicken each week, but because of legal constraints on on-farm slaughter facilities, it held off on providing this service.

Brookfield sells other locally grown items in the farm shop as a service to members. (This is where the homemade frozen yogurt comes in.) This year, Dan worked with a local dairy, Cooks Farm, that makes its own ice cream from antibiotic-free milk. Not only is there fresh, local milk, there are unbelievable treats called snackers, two chocolate chip cookies filled with vanilla ice cream. Thankfully, the children still love to pick and stuff vegetables into their mouths as much as ever.

Other items for sale include local eggs, milk and cream, sausages, medicinal and culinary herb products, honey, apples, pears, and soap. "Just Soap" is a wonderful product, manufactured by a farm member using a bicycle-powered contraption, but more importantly, it feels good to support local folk. Again, these products are provided primarily as a service to shareholders; the farm does not make a great deal of money on them. Products will vary, depending on where you live and who is producing what in your local area. Sunflower Fields Family Farm and CSA in Iowa offers these items from other producers: flowers, chickens, turkeys, beef, pork, bison, eggs, honey, bread, pies, cookies, apples, soap, and shiitake mushrooms.[5]

So you have your bags of produce, you've picked what is ready in the field, you have paid for the few extras from local growers, and you've checked your name off the list for the week. What else? Grab a newsletter and stuff it in your bag. Call your children, who are among the raspberry bushes or tomato plants, and head home.

When you get home and have put away all your goods, take a minute and read the newsletter. Most CSAs have newsletters to keep you up to date on what's been happening on the farm. Remember, you share in this enterprise. You committed up front with your financial contributions, and you might want to know how things are coming in. Is the farm suffering from a drought? How are the insects? Are there any serious problems? Does the farm need any extra help with weeding? Will your lawn leaves be helpful to the compost piles? Dan usually shares the status of certain crops, especially if they seem to be suffering in any way. In addition to the "news," members receive weekly recipes using something just harvested. These come in a handy index card size, so you can accumulate them over the years. Newsletters vary from farm to farm. Their purpose is to make a connection, and it works if you read them.

Finally, you will need menu-planning know-how. Keep those recipes from the newsletters; they will prove to be invaluable. Thankfully, as the CSA movement enlarges, the number of vegetable cookbooks is also growing. One great one comes from the Madison Area Community Supported Agriculture Coalition (MACSAC) in Wisconsin. *From Asparagus to Zucchini: A Guide to Farm-Fresh, Seasonal Produce* has been put together specifically with CSA members in mind. More than 406 different vegetable and herbs listed cover 370 recipes for those of us struggling with transforming this food from produce in the bag to dinner on the plate. Another wonderful lifesaver is RecipeSource on the web: **<www.recipesource.com>**. Clicking on "parsnips" one day gave me a long list of magic tricks for mealtimes. Finally, check out your local bookstore for cookbooks that lay out their recipes by vegetable.

Annual zucchini bake-off failure

I never seem to be able to win this thing. For goodness' sake, there aren't that many entries, although the numbers have been increasing every year. Each summer, the farm holds a zucchini bake-off potluck party. Everyone laughs about how silly it is, but I know that underneath it all, they take it as seriously as I do. Well, maybe.

One year, I came very close with my zucchini pizza. (I share the recipe below, but keep in mind, it did not win.) The only real oohs and aahs came from the homemade crust. This year, I didn't have the energy to make pizza dough, so I tried a similar concoction on pasta ... even fewer votes. I will never top farmer Karen's special family recipe for zucchini pasta, so I should give up on that.

Contest entries are numbered, and at the end of the potluck, everyone is supposed to vote for his or her favorite. I always try to influence voting by commenting on that "superb dish" to groups of four or five; or convincing my children to stuff the ballot box, but to no avail. Either my children have learned honesty too well, or I'm just not that great a campaigner.

This year's winner was a pizza, but the crust was made with zucchini. How creative is that? Even I must admit it was pretty yummy. Last year, the

Now sit down with your family and, if you are so inclined, give thanks. Our family's favorite, holding hands: "Bless this meal, bless this circle, and bless this Earth!" It is fitting that it came from the founders of our farm, David and Claire Fortier. Now, dig in ... the most memorable mouthful of morsels from the Earth. Welcome to the world of Community Supported Agriculture!

Tell me more!

If you are excited but still need more, let's look at what shareholders and others have to say. First, Jack Cooley at the University of Massachusetts researched CSAs and found the two main reasons for joining a farm were to support local farming (97 percent) and quality of produce (93 percent).[6] *The Journal of Sustainable Agriculture* winner dashed in at the last minute with a piping hot selection for dessert: zucchini brownies. Since the voting happens at the end of the meal, and Abby's dessert is always warm and yummy, it is no wonder she pulls rank.

Now for my plan ... next year, I'll arrive at dessert time with a piping hot zucchini-crusted chocolate pizza with decorative frosting "Vote for Me!" Oh, well, maybe I'd better stick to trying new recipes.

Zucchini Pizza

- Make pizza dough using any recipe. Watch your time, as it takes a while.
- Flatten the dough and cover it with the following topping:
- Sauté zucchini slices – make sure you use little ones no larger than one inch in diameter – in garlic and olive oil. (If you are not doing a zucchini bake-off entry, try using yellow squash of the same size for a bit more visual balance.) Add some basil and oregano and sauté a minute longer.
- Lay out evenly on the crust.
- Cover the zucchini mix with crumbled feta cheese and shredded mozzarella – not so much that you don't see the zucchini. Add salt and pepper to taste. Pop in the oven for 15–20 minutes at 450 degrees or just before the cheese browns.

reviewed other survey results that point clearly to the same motivations. The two main factors influencing the decision to join were the availability of fresh, organic, seasonal food, and being able to support local agriculture.[7] Results of a survey of shareholders from Winnipeg "suggest that consumer interest in the concept of CSA is a result of appealing both to the desire for good food and the desire to be part of a food system that makes sense."[8]

You probably read between the lines to understand my initial reason for joining the farm: I wanted my children to grow up respecting and eating healthier food, and I knew I wasn't modeling that behavior. Consistent with my own experience are survey results showing that people's diets changed when they became members of a farm. One study found that more than 80 percent of members said they ate more vegetables after joining a farm, with 60 percent indicating that their children did,

> "Survey results show that people's diets changed when they became members of a farm. One study found that more than 80 percent of members said they ate more vegetables after joining a farm, with 60 percent indicating that their children did, too."

too. As one respondent commented, "I have only recently become aware of the importance of fresh vegetables since joining the farm. I have learned new recipes, techniques in cooking ... I hope that by exposing my children this young to the farm ... that they will develop healthy eating habits."[9]

Some people join a farm because they know intuitively it is better to eat local and organic food, but they are not exactly sure why. As reporter David Wann wrote in the *Denver Post*, "My experience at the Cresset farm made me realize why organic produce often looks and tastes healthier than standard fare. Taste and appearance reflect the knowledge and care that go into the food."[10]

The response to CSA is visceral. It is possible to talk about what you like and dislike, but after a summer, the connection goes beyond words. *Newsday*, the daily newspaper of Long Island, New York, took a share at Golden Earthworm to learn firsthand about CSA. After 27 weeks of receiving a box full of fresh fruit and veggies, their only real frustration was a lack of ripe tomatoes. As one reporter put it, "... it was a treat to see what surprises each week brought, a challenge to base our meals on the contents of the box." Further into the article, the writers couldn't hide their true emotional attachment to the experience. They quoted another customer reassuring the farmer of her devotion: "Esther (the customer) said to the farmer, 'As long as you keep growing these vegetables, I'll keep buying them.' We [*Newsday*] will, too, with thanks in our hearts."

But I live in New York City!

If you are thinking, "That's fine for you who live near nature, but I reside in the midst of concrete," don't give up hope. One of the most organized and progressive groups in the country — Just Food — works to connect New York City residents with many different CSAs just outside the city.

Just Food is a non-profit organization founded by Kathy Lawrence in 1995 to help develop a just and sustainable food system in the New York City region. They collaborate with farmers and groups to increase availability of healthy, locally-grown food for New Yorkers, particularly those with strong emphasis on reaching out to low-income communities. One of their programs is the "CSA in NYC" program that works to make connections between community groups and farms just outside the city. They do not work as a middleman, collecting share prices or managing delivery; they simply help the two work together initially. They match farms and city groups, helping the latter to develop a distribution system. One of the earliest farms to join the program was Stoneledge Farm in South Cairo, New York. In 1996, four years after Debbie and Pete Kavakos began growing produce on an acre of land in upstate New York, they contacted Just Food to help find New York residents interested in connecting with a farm. They now provide 140 shares on 15 acres and would like to expand to 300 shares over the next three or four years.[11]

Just Food is continuing to expand its farm membership. Ruth Katz, the new executive director, mentioned to me that they are currently working with 15 core farms and 26 city groups. Their CSA program grew by more than 25 percent between 2001 and 2002.[12] Check out its website for delivery locations and farms. **<www.justfood.org>**

Similar programs are sprouting up in urban areas throughout North America. In Quebec, Equiterre has been working to connect farmers and consumers, and recently added 50 new CSA farms. In November 2000, they hosted the first Canadian CSA conference, "To Harvest, To Eat and To Share." They provide training for growers and brochures for consumers, and their website provides a map of drop-off points in the city of Montreal **<www.equiterre.qc.ca>**.

One of Equiterre's farms is Greta's Organic Gardens. Dave and Greta Kryger started their small organic farm six years ago in St. Isidore, east of Ottawa, with vegetables and a few chickens, ducks, geese, turkeys, goats, pigs, and beef cattle for their own use. Their project is now in its fourth year, and membership rose from 15 families in the first year to 85 families in 2001. They grow more than 50 varieties of vegetables, from beans to tomatillos, plus herbs, and are open to requests for additional varieties. Free-range fowl are raised on local, organically grown grains. For its CSA customers, Greta's offers organized workships on the farm (composting, herbs, etc.) and other more social events (corn roasts, barbecues, and harvest parties), as well as picnics and potluck suppers in town.

Cities are certainly serving up their share of CSA opportunities. One of the largest farms in the US is Angelic Organics, serving ten distribution sites within the city limits of Chicago, and another 12 in the Chicago suburbs. At least three farms serve at least 50 members each in Atlanta, Georgia: Strong Roots Farm in Watkinsville; Gaia Farm in East Atlanta; and Union Agricultural Institute in Blairsville.

Madison, Wisconsin, has so much interest that there is a Madison Area Community Supported Agriculture Coalition. Their goal is to provide information and educational materials for CSA members and the general public about CSA farming, sustainable agriculture and eating seasonally and locally.

What about those who can't afford it?

Organizations across the country are helping to deliver the benefits of community farming to those who cannot afford to pay. The Partner Shares program in Wisconsin, for example, aims to provide CSA shares to low-income households. In 2001, it provided matching funds for 35 CSA shares to 25 households and five agency-supported homes, to serve an estimated 380 people. The group also helped provide funding for low-income seniors wishing to join a CSA farm.[13] It is a modest beginning, maybe, but an effort nonetheless.

Just Food, described earlier in this chapter, also aims many of its programs specifically at sharing the bounty with low-income communities. Many farms across the country have developed some way of sharing with those in need. As a matter of fact, the CSA census asked farmers this very question, and 49 percent indicated they offered low-income programs for their communities. These included donations of unclaimed shares, organizing donations from shareholders, and donating a portion of the harvest to food banks. Perhaps the most popular form of low-income program was trading shares for work or barter.

One of my favorite programs is in the city of Hartford, Connecticut. The Holcomb Farm CSA project was established in 1994 by the Hartford Food System (more in Chapter 20) and the Friends of the Holcomb Farm on land donated by Tudor and Laura Holcomb and grows for 200 households and 13 community organizations. Half of its membership is made up of low-income families, and the community organizations serve another 1,000 low-income people. Cropland has increased from five to 168 acres, and production has risen from 32,000 to 120,000 pounds since its inception. It is hard to believe there is more. The farm also has a program run by the Hartford Food System, **<www.hartfordfood.org>**, a non-profit organization that tries to increase access to affordable and nutritious food, that teaches urban and minority youths about agriculture and augments their diet with produce.[14]

Build it and they shall come

No CSA near you? Go ahead and get your closest friends, congregation, or book club, find a grower, and start your own. If this sounds a bit overwhelming, remember, many have come before you. Just think of the Ottawa Organic Food Alternative (OOFA) that started in 1988 with four city folks figuring out the veggie requirements of ten families. In their first spring, 20 families were sharing the foodstuffs; by the end of harvest, they had 40 families. Ten years later, 80 families share the fare of 20 local producers who provide the basics, plus more unusual items, such as goat milk, soy products, hempseed cookies, and wild rice.

It helps if you live in one of the urban locations that have CSA support groups, like Just Food, aiming to connect you to a grower. If not, you might want to try the new Robyn VanEn Center, located at Wilson College in Chambersburg, Pennsylvania. Its website **<www.csacenter.org>** provides a great deal of information and contacts. It maintains the national database for all CSAs (finding the CSA farm nearest you) and will answer inquiries and provide relevant materials. Another new addition to the CSA world is the biennial conference, which the Center co-sponsors. Attend one of these popular events and you'll meet the many participants of this exciting movement. The center will have the details on its website.

The must-have manual, however, to starting a CSA is *Sharing the Harvest* by Elizabeth Henderson, a veteran CSA farmer, with Robyn VanEn. Elizabeth and Robyn were in the early stages of developing the book when Robyn's untimely death occurred. Elizabeth ultimately did a magnificent job of covering the entire movement, with numerous examples and how-to worksheets. The manual provides such useful information as sample budgets, legal structures, equipment lists, job descriptions, planning charts, and what should be included in a share. Her "Steps to Forming a CSA" outline is just a morsel of the many details you will want to consider. Check out page 34 of her book for the complete steps.

A Canadian graduate student, Amunda Salm, interviewed CSA producers in the vicinity of Ottawa and Southern Ontario. From those surveys, she developed eight suggestions for farmers starting a CSA operation:

- Talk to other CSA farmers
- Start small
- Be prepared to work very hard
- Try to set up a core group
- Research the consumer base in the area
- Depend on many marketing outlets
- Try to carry on through the winter
- Cooperate with other farmers

WEBSITE

For further information, check out the Ecological Agriculture Projects website at McGill University **<www.eap.mcgill.ca>**.

Once you have your core group, your farmer, and the details in place and you want a bit more technical help before the first seeds sink into the soil, a few excellent CSA farmers, including our own farmer Dan, are running a fee-based consulting group, CSA Works. They can provide examples of materials and assess your readiness to hit the dirt. Alternatively, more Land Grant universities are providing services to CSAs through Cooperative Extension.

Just remember, you *can* do it. There are plenty of people who want to help and see you succeed. It *will* help change the world!

Is CSA really the answer to future farming?

Some give a resounding "Yes!" CSA provides a unique relationship between consumer and farmer, one that takes away the middlemen, the packaging, the processing, and the mystery of what it takes to raise food. It shares the risk of crop failure directly with the end user instead of using tax dollars for relief programs.

CSA cuts down on the waste created by the market economy. For example, a commercial vegetable grower in Columbia County, New York, found that he wasted about 30 percent of his harvest every year because of fluctuating market demand (quantity) and food that didn't meet market standards (quality), such as appearance and size.[15] CSA shares the harvest equally, and when there are leftovers, farms have either a donation procedure or the produce ends up in compost, working its way back to the fields the next year.

CSA saves valuable open land in all sorts of locations, close to urban and suburban residents. One farm in Santa Barbara, California, shows in its brochure an aerial photograph of the land years ago, when it was simply one of many other fields; today, it is surrounded by homes. In a place like Massachusetts, where very little farmland is left, CSA holds the promise of maintaining a few more vistas, a handful of cows to pass on the way to work, and small tractors putzing along the road, ensuring a more manageable speed limit for all.

CSA creates the need for on-farm diversity, since farm families want all sorts of different foods, not just one. It addresses many of the concerns we've read about throughout this book. It is as close as we know right now to solving the myriad of problems attached to today's agriculture. Most experts say we cannot change the world with the concept. I say we can. I don't believe everyone will change over to the

CSA model; that would be a fantasy beyond dreams. I do believe, however, that as more people become aware of the alternative, more people will reduce their tolerance for our sickened food system. I believe in the power of consumers to make change, to rise up in their own individual ways. We, as eaters, have a right to share the Earth's bounty, grown with attention and care.

> "I believe in the power of consumers to make change, to rise up in their own individual ways."

18

Who's Got Time to Cook?

IF "DO-IT-YOURSELF" WENT OUT THE WINDOW ALONG WITH AN ABUNDANCE OF TIME, you can still call yourself an eco-eater by choosing an environmentally friendly restaurant. We are fortunate today to have the Chef's Collaborative and some other exciting projects in the eco-dining area. If you, too, want to dine "green," there are ways of encouraging your favorite chef to buy local and to think sustainable.

Chefs do it

In *Food & Wine Magazine*'s 1997 Chef's Survey, administered by Louis Harris & Associates, 76 percent of those chefs surveyed responded "Yes" to the question, "Do you actively seek out organically grown ingredients?" According to the National Restaurant Association, organic items are now offered by about 57 percent of restaurants with per-person dinner checks of $25 or more. In addition, 29 percent of restaurants with prices in the $15 to $24 range also offer organic items. This is very good news. More and more of our entrees are being prepared with the Earth in mind.

We read about one of the leaders of the environmental food choices movement in Chapter 7. Alice Waters, renowned chef and partner of Chez Panisse in Berkeley,

California, has influenced many to change their habits to eco-dining. Part of her message was quoted in the preface to the *Green Kitchen Handbook*: "Food can be transformative in everyone's life … How you eat and how you choose your food is an act that combines the political — your place in the world — with the most intensely personal — the way you use your mind and your senses, together for the gratification of your soul."[1] Chez Panisse opened its doors in 1971 and has been a model for fine dining, with the Earth in mind ever since. The restaurant was the first to hire a full-time "forager," whose job is to find local, organic, or sustainable foods and to build relationships with their suppliers.

> "I have enormous gratitude for Alice Waters and all those chefs who have labored to create a cornucopia of flavors and freshness with gifts from the Earth."

I have enormous gratitude for Alice Waters and all those chefs who have labored to create a cornucopia of flavors and freshness with gifts from the Earth. When I first began to experiment with more healthy, wholesome foods, I found my creations tasted as if they should have been served to bunnies and ponies instead of people. Dry greens and heavy, whole-wheat dishes screamed, "Don't eat me!" Thankfully, before I became too frustrated, recipes began to emerge from top restaurants around the country that filled my previous "pet foods" with flavors beyond my hopes and dreams.

Another West Coast restaurant dedicated to local, sustainable cuisine is the Peerless Restaurant in Ashland, Oregon. An interview by GlobalChefs, an on-line magazine, captured the essence of this creative process. "The basic premise of cooking is to always start with the freshest, highest-quality ingredients and to then coax and encourage the best out of them."[2]

On the opposite coast, Judy Wicks of the White Dog Café in Philadelphia is spreading her version of the importance of eco-dining and advocacy. As she described on the cover of her newsletter in the summer of 2001, "As part of a commitment to support our local economy and help preserve Pennsylvania's agricultural landscape, we anticipate purchasing 80 percent of our food from local farmers this summer." The restaurant is a hub of activity, hosting public issue table talks and storytelling, community tours, and a variety of diverse and seasonal parties.

Wicks and other chefs throughout the country have not only modeled sustainable behavior at their own establishments, they have created a movement for tremendous change through a single national voice, the Chef's Collaborative.

The Chef's Collaborative

In July 1993, an educational initiative began at Oldways Preservation and Exchange Trust (a Boston-based non-profit organization focused on healthy eating) that would encourage chefs to use their restaurants as pulpits for good-for-Earth foods. To quote its fact sheet, "The Chef's Collaborative is a national network of more than 1,000 members of the food community who promote sustainable cuisine by celebrating the joys of local, seasonal and artisinal cooking".[3]

> "The Chef's Collaborative is a national network of more than 1,000 members of the food community who promote sustainable cuisine by celebrating the joys of local, seasonal and artisinal cooking."

Headquartered in Cambridge, Massachusetts, the Chef's Collaborative has extended its influence to chefs around the country with a statement of principles and a charge to further the movement. Today they hold annual conferences, seminars, and tastings; publish position papers and chef's guides; and send out newsletters and communiqués to inform their collective.

Originally interested in the sources of their produce, the Collaborative's current focus is on seafood. Remember the issues discussed in Chapter 12, "A Fishy Story"? The chefs' group is spearheading the movement to change menus to include sustainable types of seafood. As reported in the *Seattle Times*, "According to a study by the Stanford Graduate School of Business, two-thirds of seafood sold in America is through restaurants. While much of that is through informal eateries such as McDonald's or Red Lobster, about half is prepared and served by white-tablecloth restaurants."[4]

Clearly, we have a hard time keeping on top of the facts about our fish. The Audubon wallet card can help at the grocery, but remembering to ask about the source of your dining-out dishes can be difficult. If restaurants are modeling the behavior by choosing appropriate fare, this can truly help us all. Hopefully, it will also catch on at some of the other "informal eateries" that have a big influence on the net loss of our underwater kingdom.

The Chef's Collaborative Seafood Solutions campaign includes workshops for chefs around the country, in addition to information-sharing through literature and guides. "Chefs are the gatekeepers of the food industry," said Mike Sutton, director of marine conservation for the David and Lucille Packard Foundation. (The Foundation is one of the country's largest private philanthropic organizations, and is funding the $200,000 campaign.)[5]

This seems like such a wonderful effort. I have always believed the Chef's Collaborative was one of the shining lights of the sustainable agriculture movement. It came as a great shock that there could be a group unhappy with their efforts. A short article in the *Denver Post* in the winter of 2001 reported on a 12-page mailing by Guest Choice Network, a coalition of 30,000 restaurateurs, which claimed, "the CC is a politically motivated group trying to abolish the consumption of meat and modern farming techniques — and return to organic farming. Guest Choice claims "the movement does not necessarily produce superior, safer, better-tasting, or healthier food — just more expensive food." A representative of the Chef's Collaborative responded, "I'm not a vegetarian, and we don't have any hidden agenda. I just want good, healthy food."[6] Apparently, so does *Gourmet* magazine, which named the nearly 100 percent organic Chez Panisse the country's best restaurant in the fall of 2001.

Other chefs' organizations are doing great work throughout North America. In Canada, Organic Advocates — Knives & Forks (kitchen knives and pitchforks) was founded in 1989 by chefs Jamie Kennedy and Michael Stadtlander. Primarily a farmer-chef group, they also hold the well-known fundraising event, Feast of Fields, which pays for a variety of projects, including *The Consumer's Guide to Eating Organics*. To order the book and access a wealth of information and valuable links, check out **<www.organicadvocates.org>**.

The Earth Pledge Foundation in New York City is doing a number of remarkable activities around sustainable cuisine. Founded in 1991, Earth Pledge focuses on sustainable activities, including foods. Since 1995, it has held dinners prepared with local and organic ingredients, as well as conducting hands-on cooking classes in its Center for Sustainable Cuisine. The organization has also put together *Sustainable Cuisine White Papers*, a collection of 40 essays from a variety of leaders in the field. The organization defines sustainable cuisine as "a derivative of sustainable development which celebrates the pleasures of food and the diversity of cultures, while recognizing the impact of food on our health and our environment. It preserves culinary traditions and addresses the need to safely nourish a growing world population."[7]

> "The Earth Pledge Foundation in New York City is doing a number of remarkable activities around sustainable cuisine."

At the end of 2001, Earth Pledge launched a feast of information for the state of New York on its website, **<www.farmtotable.org>**. Packed with delectable treats from fruit varieties, to farmer profiles, to events listings, the site is for consumers, chefs, farmers, and anyone else interested in eco-foods. The website is supposed to be the first of many to come, each focused on a different state. That would be a fabulous gift. It is one of the best sites I have ever seen.

A statewide group in our neighborhood is the Vermont Fresh Network (VFN). Through this network, more than 110 chefs have formed 250 "handshake agreements" with more than 90 farmers throughout the state.[8] To join as a producer or food business, partner members must agree to a certain number of "handshakes:" commitments to buy, instead of formal written agreements. The network then promotes both the farms and the restaurants, and partners can use the VFN logo to communicate their commitment to diners. Vermont Fresh Network holds events, produces a newsletter, and handles a variety of projects, including a "Fresh Sheet" that provides chefs with a weekly listing of available Vermont farm products.

A similar pilot project is under way as part of the Finger Lakes Culinary Bounty in New York State. In this case, the handshake agreements go beyond making purchases to actually promoting local farm products on the menus. As with the Vermont program, restaurants are then promoted as participants. These kinds of arrangements are such win-win propositions, especially for us, the consumers. I am always grateful to learn which restaurants are participating in our sustainable future.

What about eco-foods for lunch?

Remembering to eat eco-foods at restaurants is no easy affair. Here I am in the midst of writing a book on the subject, and today at lunch with a friend, I ordered a barbecued pork sandwich. What is up with that? I can almost guarantee that pig did not live a fair life. I preach ad nauseum to friends and neighbors about the importance of free-range meats, and yet without thinking of what I was eating until the fourth bite, I found myself an instant hypocrite. Thankfully, my friend reminded me of the waste of energy in self-flagellation and suggested the three-point plan, "Stop, That, Now!" I will just have to be more careful next time.

Thankfully, another friend a few hours north of here has big plans for a chain of restaurants that could help save the day. Tod Murphy is carrying the message by building a solution to our everyday dining-out problems. The Farmers' Diner is going to be amazing! Eighty percent of the food sold by the diner will be grown and/or raised within 50 miles of the restaurant. No longer would I have to worry about the pig's life on my barbecue sandwich. The animals will have been raised locally, and the farmer's practices will be transparent. In addition to the local aspect, Tod has certain environmental and social requirements, such as no use of antibiotics or hormones, and access to outdoors and pasture for animals. He hopes to further the Farmers' Diner's mission by selling the diner's products in retail outlets, further helping out the local farmers. This is good stuff. Look for Tod's prototype in Barre, Vermont, and then pray for one near you.

The Farmers' Diner is not the only everyday food operation trying to stick with sustainable values. Thankfully, more and more are under conversion from conventional to sustainable menu items. David Yudkin of Hot Lips Pizza in Portland, Oregon, competes with the chain pizzerias and yet maintains his dedication to sourcing local and seasonal foods. Voicing his desire to be a leader in responsible business, Yudkin has stated that local produce accounts for 25 percent of his food budget, and in the summer, this increases to 60 percent.[9]

Can fast foods be eco-foods?

What do we do about fast food? Eric Schlosser, author of *Fast Food Nation: The dark side of the all-American meal*, says, "Don't buy it!" But, we do, to the tune of $112 billion in the year 2000.[10] I have always felt, intuitively, that fast food was not good for my family, but I had never gone through the effort to do the fact-finding. To be honest, faced with running from piano lessons to sports practice, squeezing in homework and my own work, hurried stops at fast-food joints seemed unavoidable. I love to cook. I love to make my own granola, breads, salsas, pizzas, etc. I am also too busy ... a lot. If I found out what might exist beyond the fast-food façade, I was afraid I would be forced to change.

And then along comes a book that does the fact-finding for us, no holds barred. After reading *Fast Food Nation*, you may find your conscience, like mine, severely compromised the next time you stop at a fast-food restaurant. The stories are overwhelming. Schlosser wakes us up to a myriad of labor issues, to the level of impact the fast-food chains have on how our food is raised, and to the almost non-food aspect of our orders. In the book's epilogue, Schlosser reminds us of our collective power to do something:

> The first step toward meaningful change is by far the easiest: stop buying it. The executives who run the fast food industry are not bad men. They are businessmen.

They will sell free-range, organic, grass-fed hamburgers if you demand it. They will sell whatever sells at a profit. The usefulness of the market, its effectiveness as a tool, cuts both ways. The real power of the American consumer has not yet been unleashed. The heads of Burger King, KFC, and McDonald's should feel daunted; they're outnumbered. There are three of them and almost three hundred million of you. A good boycott, a refusal to buy, can speak much louder than words. Sometimes the more irresistible force is the most mundane.[11]

So what can the over-committed soccer mom do? Don't worry — Gary Hirshberg and a handful of others are coming to the rescue. If you have heard of Gary Hirshberg before, it was probably as the founder of Stonyfield Farm, the well-known successful yogurt maker who serves up organic versions. Now Gary has taken on another project. When he told me about it at the 2001 Natural Products Expo, I gave a sigh of relief. Finally — a fast eco-foods restaurant! That is it in a nutshell.

"Finally — a fast eco-foods restaurant!"

O'Naturals opened in May 2001 in Falmouth, Maine. The company plans three more stores on the East Coast in the next two years. So far, the restaurant is generating sales of about $100,000 a month, comparable to the monthly sales of a typical McDonald's franchise.[12] This is very exciting. I reviewed the on-line menu and found Alaskan salmon (the only version that falls in the green category on the Audubon card), local potatoes, and plenty of organic items. The children's items would certainly appeal to my kids. I will be very grateful when this option becomes available near me.

Gary's comments to a *New York Times* reporter covering the restaurant's opening hit very close to home. "A lot of people eat at fast-food restaurants begrudgingly … they buy healthy, low-fat, natural, and organic foods at the grocery store, but they really have no choice when they're out on the highway or in a hurry and the Golden Arches is all there is."[13]

In addition to this bit of good news come reports that similar restaurants are popping up across the country. Heartwise Express serves wraps and noodle bowls, salads, soups and veggie burgers in downtown Chicago, with plans to open two more soon. Pret a Manger, the UK sandwich chain, has just opened a handful of shops in New York City. Pret a Manger sells 300,000 chemical-free gourmet sandwiches a day through its 106 outlets, makes its food from scratch, refuses to use additives, and chooses only high-quality, non-GMO, organic ingredients. Its chickens are free-range birds from Spain.[14] News is that McDonald's purchased a one-third stake in the chain. "What does this mean?" you might ask. We'll just have to wait and see. For now, suffice it to say that we may just get it our way.

Take the cheerleader out to eat

Another opportunity to practice that cheer … let's have eco-foods here! You may not don bobby socks and saddle shoes, but expressing your appreciation for organic or local menu items sends the word back to the kitchen. Ask your waiter about the source of the tomatoes, and when he says, "I dunno," scrunch up your face and give a big disappointed pout. Next, ask if the fish falls in the safety zone for sustainability. After he trots back from the kitchen, send him off to find out which grain is organic. And for the grand finale, ask if the cream on the raspberries comes from rBGH-free cows. By the time you get the order in, your chef will get the message. She'll be signing up for next year's Chef's Collaborative conference.

> "Expressing your appreciation for organic or local menu items sends the word back to the kitchen. Ask your waiters about the source of the tomatoes, and when he says, I dunno, scrunch up your face and give a big disappointed pout."

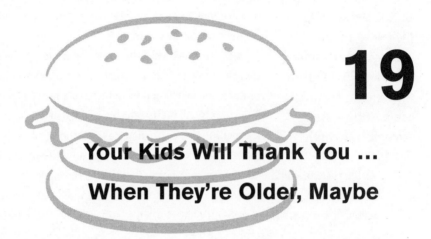

19

Your Kids Will Thank You ...
When They're Older, Maybe

SOME SCHOOLS AND COLLEGES ARE BRINGING ECO-EATING TO THEIR MENUS. Change that cafeteria food — tell your child's administrator, "Go green!" "Out of" the mouths of babes may be "into" in this case. More and more schools are serving their students right by adding organics and other natural foods to their menus and adding composting to their ecological strengths. This little step is particularly courageous in light of new fast-food marketing aimed at our schools.

Fast food in their face

They call it cradle-to-grave marketing, and the target is our children. No fewer than five multinational corporations run "school programs," some more educationally oriented than others, but still promoting their products. Have you ever had your daughter come home with a coupon for pizza because she read enough books that week? Now try to say "no" to a family meal out to redeem that coupon, which, by the way, will force you and the rest of the family to buy a meal you wouldn't have otherwise.

According to a *New York Times* review of a report from the General Accounting Office last fall, "Some marketing professionals are increasingly targeting children in schools, companies are becoming known for their success in negotiating contracts between school districts and beverage companies, and both educators and corporate managers are attending conferences to learn how to increase revenue from in-school marketing for their schools and companies."[1]

> "More and more schools are serving their students right by adding organics and other natural foods to their menus and adding composting to their ecological strengths."

It is one thing when the audiovisual equipment has been donated by a big food company, and quite another when brand name fast food is introduced into the school cafeteria. The latter is still pretty rare, but enough of a concern to keep a watchful eye, particularly as childhood obesity hits all-time highs. *Time* magazine carried an article (January 2002) on the issue of childhood obesity, specifically pointing to the subject of corporate products in our schools as one of the culprits: "... hundreds of cash-strapped school districts around the country have turned to soft-drink bottlers, who offer as much as $100,000 a year for exclusive 'pouring' contracts to place vending machines in school hallways. Principals have opened their cafeterias to such fast-food franchises as Taco Bell and Burger King. 'If your task was to make the American child as unhealthy as possible, could you do much better than fast food and soft drinks in the cafeterias?' asks Kelly Brownell, a psychologist at Yale University."[2]

Thankfully, my children's school has so far been spared. But overseeing of their school lunch choices is still very difficult. When my children report how they figured out how to forego the day's beans or supplement their dessert with ice cream, I freak out. No big surprise that I don't hear those stories anymore. Does that mean it doesn't happen? Doubtful. My children certainly don't find their lunchboxes full of snacks and sugary items from home, so school grounds probably present a haven of possibilities.

The *Time* article brings us up to date on obesity. "According to the latest federal figures, the percentage of youngsters ages 6 to 11 who are overweight has tripled since the 1960s, to 13 percent. As many as one in seven kids is obese, and doctors are seeing dangerously obese children as young as age two. Last month the Surgeon General issued an urgent call for the nation to fight its growing weight problem, a move that was sparked in part by the epidemic rates of childhood obesity. Overweight children are more than twice as likely to have high blood pressure or heart disease as children of normal weight. Even more alarming is the number of children with Type 2, or non-insulin-dependent, diabetes."[3]

Thankfully, this national epidemic has brought recognition of the issue of school food to a national level. At the start of 2001, the USDA provided a report to Congress, "Foods Sold in Competition with USDA School Meal Programs" which outlines various recommendations to combat the commercial alternatives to nutritious foods in schools. The report states, "While studies indicate that the school meal programs do contribute to better nutrition and healthier eating behaviors for children who participate, competitive foods undermine the nutrition integrity of the programs and discourage participation."[4]

I don't know if I could say school lunches are healthy or nutritious. One piece of insight I would rather have not had to ingest was a short excerpt from the book *Fast Food Nation* in which the author details the substandard quality of meat purchased by the national school lunch program. Testing for Salmonella and *E. coli* on our children's foods has, thankfully, caught quite a bit of contaminated meat over the years.[5] However, we may have to keep a close eye on the continuation of those safeguards. In the spring of 2001, the *New York Times* carried a story headlined, "US Proposes End to Testing for Salmonella in School Beef," in which it reported the Bush administration had proposed dropping the tests.[6]

From the large-scale advertising messages to the small-scale bacteria, it seems our schools may need a hand from us in safeguarding our young.

Hooray for the heroes!

And then there are those who are making change. Some schools have guts ... and should be commended for it. Some schools are kicking out the corporations, others are investing in improved nutritional programs, and many are turning to their local farmers for their lunchtime fare. Others are unbelievably creative, connecting gardening, cooking, and lunchtime feasts. Some of these programs are so good, you may just want to move your family there!

Let's start with elementary and high schools. California

> "Some schools are kicking out the corporations, others are investing in improved nutritional programs, and many are turning to their local farmers for their lunchtime fare."

seems to be one of the lead states in developing a connection between the school cafeteria and the farm. Farmer's Market Salad Bar, a pilot program that began in one of Santa Monica's schools in 1997, seems to have kick-started a national farm-to-school program. The Santa Monica program, which has now spread throughout the district and is moving into Los Angeles, was originally organized by the Occidental

Community Food Security Project. Produce for a daily salad bar in the cafeterias is purchased twice weekly at a local farmers' market.

At a similar project at Pioneer Elementary School in Davis, California, the program is referred to as the "Crunch Lunch" salad bar option. One third-grader gave the program a dream endorsement: "Crunch lunch rocks! I want to eat it every day!" The option includes six to eight seasonal vegetables and fruits, and two or three protein-rich foods, such as eggs, tuna, fish, beans, and turkey. The program is supplemented with a gardening curriculum, composting and recycling activities, and tours of local farms.[7]

Some of the farm-to-school programs are simple, such as in North Carolina, where the state legislature gave grants to schools to buy local farm products. In the Florida Panhandle, a program was initiated by a small group of farmers who organized into the New North Florida Cooperative. This group developed a solid relationship with a couple of local schools' food service directors by regularly providing quality fresh-cut greens plus watermelons, strawberries, blackberries, and grapes.

The program "From Farm to School: Improving Small Farm Viability and School Meals," funded by a $2 million grant from the USDA Initiative for Future Agriculture and Food Systems, has now expanded to include 19 projects in California, New Jersey, and New York. There are other pilot projects in Connecticut, North Carolina, Kentucky, and Florida.[8]

One of the earliest projects and possibly the first to go beyond a salad bar and provide entire meal selections is in Berkeley, California, where the program also directed that genetically altered and irradiated foods be removed from their offerings. The school district decided that one way to get fresh food into its cafeterias, in addition to buying from nearby farmers, was to grow its own crops. Students help grow their own food by working in the school district's organic garden, and 11 of Berkeley's 16 schools have their own gardens. The Edible School Yard at Martin Luther King Jr. Middle School incorporates planting, gardening, harvesting, cooking, and eating to teach children the entire process of food production.[9]

> **"There is nothing like a garden for an educational tool; no manufactured alternatives can beat the awe-inspiring bounty of nature."**

There is nothing like a garden for an educational tool; no manufactured alternatives can beat the awe-inspiring bounty of nature. This spring my children planted their first "wholly-owned" gardens. Time after time, they would rush indoors to show me the fruits of their labors. "Look, Mom, it's a real bean!" ...

or a tiny green tomato, or a first squash flower. And each time, the excitement was all-consuming. You might think after more than a handful of these experiences, it would wane slightly. No, here they'd come, flying into the house, "Look, Mom ..." I think all the carrots I was treated to measured under a quarter-inch long. In an article in *Gastronomica* about children playing in the garden, Laura De Lind writes, "Unlike 'hatching' dinosaurs or sucking yogurt from a Mylar tube, our physical engagement in the puzzling and time-consuming process of raising vegetables or flowers, of building insect habitats or soil, can be a source of personal satisfaction and meaningful work."[10]

So many schools are jumping into school-ground gardens and farm visits, but not nearly so many model the behavior of eating from Mother Earth. The programs that make the connection give me real faith that the link won't be lost and that children will grow up with more than a milk-comes-from-a-carton mentality. This sentiment is confirmed in a report published in *Farming Alternatives* in 2001. "By linking the cafeteria to nutrition and sustainable agriculture education in the classroom, and to farm visits and hands-on experiences growing food in school gardens, schools are incorporating an experiential approach with the potential to transform children's eating habits."[11]

Exciting connections are being made in a number of schools in Santa Fe, New Mexico. A pilot program, Local Harvest, is teaming up with a renowned multicultural food education program, Cooking with Kids. This educational program, developed by Lynn Walters and inspired by research from Cornell University's Dr. Antonia Demas, involves tasting and cooking culturally diverse foods and special cafeteria meal selections a couple of times a month. The program's design is meant to improve children's nutrition by increasing acceptance of nutritious foods.

You may be ready to pack your bags and move your children closer to one of these wonderful opportunities, but it may be more effective to consider something similar at home. As the *Time* magazine article suggested, "Parents can influence what their children like to eat. Kids are born with a sweet tooth and a salty one, but they have to learn to enjoy other tastes. They often need repeated introductions to such healthy fare as beans and other veggies."[12]

Let's go to college

When I think of colleges and new food choices, I think of my stepson at Boston University. I was never very successful at expanding his taste buds when he was younger; I was still stuck in my fettuccini Alfredo stage. During his freshman year, he found himself hating the fast-food options in the student union and wanting to expand his culinary repertoire to healthier foods. So he set out to learn to cook in his basement dorm kitchen. Not a very long-lived experience, it was still self-motivated and seems important to him to this day. I think he has also been convinced by meals at home (and my long diatribes) that locally grown, in-season, and organic foods are tastier and better for us all.

Thankfully, on the college level there is already more awareness of sustainability issues and the need to eat with the environment in mind. Some campuses now provide naturally and ecologically grown products in their regular menus, not just in their alternative student-run cooperatives. It often starts with veggie burgers and expands to locally grown fruits and vegetables.

One of the pioneer efforts began in 1986 at Hendrix College in Conway, Arkansas. At that time, students conducted a study, gathering information on the sources of the food served at that college. The students learned that 93 percent of the sources were outside of the Arkansas area, most often California and Mexico. With help from a local non-profit organization, Meadowcreek, the college was able to increase its use of local food from 7 percent to 30 percent in three years, resulting in more than $200,000 being spent on local food each year.[13]

The University of Wisconsin also connects local growers to campus food service on a number of its campuses. In 1998, the UW Madison's Center for Integrated Agricultural Systems supported a preliminary study of the potential for colleges and universities across the country to purchase locally grown, sustainable foods, and since has helped to pilot these programs throughout the state.

I remember speaking five years ago with a professor of sustainable agriculture at the hip, progressive college in our town. (With five colleges here, they all have their reputations.) Many of the students had been working to integrate local foods in their dining halls, but were bumping up against the college's large food-service contractor. Many dining services are managed by these outside companies that have been directed to purchase in bulk from their own internal sources. Instead of local, seasonal fare, the food is shipped in from a central warehouse in a location suitable for the company, not necessarily for the school. Campuses have found a number of such barriers, and these pilot projects are working hard to develop solutions so all students can enjoy eco-foods.

> "Some of the programs are brewing because of a much larger commitment to sustainability."

Some of the programs are brewing because of a much larger commitment to sustainability. A real effort is being made on many campuses to model the same messages students are hearing in the classrooms about stewardship of our Earth. In the late 1980s, leaders in academic ecology came together in Talloires, France, and developed a set of principles calling on higher education institutions to set an example in their day-to-day campus operations in all matters of environmental concern.[14] More than 250 colleges and universities, including 50 in America, voluntarily signed and agreed to the principles. Sustainability projects have been popping up on campuses ever since, aimed at integrating recycling, locally and sustainably grown food services, IPM practices on school grounds, curriculum, architectural and building plans, and myriad other activities.

> "Leading a parade down the center of town may not be necessary to get your school administrator to consider your eco-eating requests. Simple steps can start a whole new menu."

How to be a squeaky wheel

Let's say you want to help your school be a model. Leading a parade down the center of town may not be necessary to get your school administrator to consider your eco-eating requests. Simple steps can start a whole new menu. If you're not a noisemaker, encouraging other parents or local farmers may be a better tactic. Since the USDA has gotten in on the act, resources may be available through its website. If not, the Community Food Security Coalition has a number of publications to encourage you. Find out more at **<www.foodsecurity.org>**.

One of the coalition's publications, *Healthy Farms, Healthy Kids*, describes seven pilot projects and provides information on some of the barriers and opportunities associated with developing such programs. Many of the pilot projects mentioned in this chapter will also be submitting reports on their work, adding to the arsenal of how-to hints for local foods-in-schools advocates. To those who lead us, and our children, to a better food system ... thank you.

20

People Helping People

MANY OF THE "GOOD" PROJECTS AND ORGANIZATIONS ARE NOT REPRESENTED on the grocery shelves. Some of these groups are dedicated to making a connection between consumers and small local farmers, while others focus on supporting the small farmers. Other organizations are teaching our children about growing food in a sustainable manner. And finally, many have taken on the bigger issues, from policy research and advocacy to farmland conservation. People who fill the offices of these (usually) shoestring-budget operations dedicate their lives to changing how we obtain our daily bread. We need to take any opportunity we can to support them beyond our food dollars, from volunteering to making donations, or even attending events.

A real movement is going on behind the scenes, one I have had the good fortune of stepping into during the past several years. I wouldn't even begin to try to name it. It has such a breadth of energies bubbling on all sorts of different levels and working on such varied solutions that I wouldn't be able to capture its essence into a single name. Elizabeth Henderson provides a great description in the book *Hungry for Profit*: "Populist in spirit, with strong feelings for civil rights and social justice, and an underlying spirituality, this movement is not linked with any political party or religious sect. It is firmly grounded in every region in the country, encompassing organic and low-input farmers; food, farming, farmworker, community food security, and hunger organizations; animal rights activists; and environmental, consumer, and religious groups."[1] Although describing each group and what it does would take a whole other book, here is a handful of examples I have not yet mentioned.

Making connections

Future Harvest: A Chesapeake Alliance for Sustainable Agriculture (CASA) is one of the first I think of as an example of regionally focused, sustainable agriculture advocacy organizations. One reason may be that I always seem to cross paths with the friendly and upbeat executive director, Bruce Mertz, at meetings and conferences. Another reason is that CASA was one of the projects funded by the Integrated Farming Systems (IFS) initiative of the Kellogg Foundation. The Kellogg Foundation has been an integral donor to many of the groups in the movement. In the first phase of the IFS program, Kellogg supported 18 community-based collaborative projects with $15 million. In the second phase, the foundation contributed $16 million to 24 organizations. As Bruce from CASA mentioned to me over the phone, "Kellogg has been responsible for the start-up of a lot of these kinds of organizations, ours being one of them." As important as the funding has been, a majority of the projects mentioned in this chapter are not actually Kellogg grant recipients. Other sustainable agriculture donors across the country include the Joyce Foundation, the Jessie Smith Noyes Foundation, and Farm Aid.

> "Future Harvest: A Chesapeake Alliance for Sustainable Agriculture (CASA) is one of the first I think of as an example of regionally focused, sustainable agriculture advocacy organizations."

CASA is a network of farmers, agricultural professionals, landowners, and consumers from the Chesapeake region. In addition to its annual conference, CASA puts out a regular newsletter and a number of "how-to" publications, and maintains a variety of directories for consumers. It has recently compiled eight publications in a series, "Small Farm Successes: Profiles of Rural Innovations," and distributed them throughout the area. One project, Amazing Grazing, resulted in *A Consumer's Guide to Grass-based Farm Products*. After reading Chapter 11, you might agree this is a much-needed resource for those looking to avoid factory-farmed meat products.

Some of the organizations that connect farmers to consumers also support local farmers with farm-based education programs. The Pennsylvania Association for Sustainable Agriculture (PASA) does this, and also spends a great deal of energy on its Community FARM (Farm Alliance for Regional Markets) initiative.

PASA activities also include a farmer-to-chef network encouraging and smoothing the way for more local foods in area restaurants; producer-only farmers' markets; the development of a "Buy Local" campaign; endorsement and support of community-supported agriculture; and facilitation of value-added projects. Value-added projects increase the value of basic foodstuffs — for example, berries could be made into pies, milk into ice cream, or meat and vegetables into stews. One value-added project is the Pennsylvania Family Farm Beef Cooperative, a network of beef producers collaboratively marketing value-added beef products (that are also antibiotic- and hormone-free) to local restaurants. PASA coordinated activities among graziers, packers, and restaurant owners to get this project started. Another of its projects is a farmer-directed dairy venture.

In addition to all its great work, PASA has gained a reputation for hosting a wonderful conference every winter. Renowned for its motivating speakers and interesting subjects, the PASA conference is a great gift to those trying to make change.

The Regional Farm & Food Project is based in Albany, New York, and encourages connections in a ten-county area around that city. Executive Director Tracy Frisch is a very active and energetic contributor to the sustainable agriculture movement. The non-profit membership organization promotes a variety of opportunities for consumers to connect with local farmers such as farm tours, workshops, open houses, community forums, harvest dinners and a quarterly newsletter. It also airs a monthly radio show on a local station. One of its programs is "Linking Children with Agriculture," which networks farmers and educators to create enhanced learning opportunities. Like PASA, it, too, has been working with local dairies, in this case to develop specialty cheeses and farm-bottled milk.

I know I am dating myself, but I remember the milkman. Once a week, we would leave the farm's empty milk bottles in the silver milk box with a note for the next delivery. I can still see it ... the milkman would arrive with his silver metal crate, collect the used bottles, and fill our cooler with the new ones. Most often it would just be milk (if I was really lucky, chocolate milk), but on occasion, Mom would ask for cottage cheese. Many of these value-added items left dairy farming when

> "PASA activities also include a farmer-to-chef network encouraging and smoothing the way for more local foods in area restaurants; producer-only farmers' markets; the development of a "Buy Local" campaign; endorsement and support of community-supported agriculture; and facilitation of value-added projects."

processing plants took over. Today, thanks to groups like Tracy's and to creative farmers themselves, farm-processed items are popping up again.

Assisting farmers with the development of value-added products has become a primary activity for some groups. The Appalachian Center for Economic Networks (ACEnet), created in 1985, is a community economic development organization based in southeastern Ohio. By 1993, ACEnet had begun investing in the specialty food sector, raising funds and constructing a licensed facility where entrepreneurs could rent the use of ovens, stoves, and food-processing equipment to produce foodstuffs. Similar programs include the Adirondack Kitchen in upstate New York, the Foodworks Culinary Center in Arcata, California, and the Food Development Centre in Manitoba, Canada.

Helping farmers

Helping farmers to reach new markets through accessible, value-added resources is just the beginning of the cornucopia of farmer-assistance projects dotting the countryside. The New England Small Farm Institute (NESFI), located in Belchertown, Massachusetts, is a beehive of farmer-support activities. I first got wind of what NESFI was doing while working for UMass Extension. Time after time, NESFI would emerge as either a leader or a collaborator in projects or programs. I have since become more involved as a member of NESFI's board of trustees, and I continue to be impressed by the number of projects it manages.

NESFI, a non-profit organization started in 1977, promotes the increased and sustainable use of the region's agricultural resources, and provides educational support and advocacy for New England's small farms. Under the direction of Judy Gillan and Kathy Ruhf, its programming and staffing have expanded, while maintaining its core focus on beginning farmers, and on sustainable small-scale agriculture. Its Small Farm Development Center library includes one of the largest specialized collections on small-scale farming and sustainable agriculture in the US. NESFI manages an apprentice-matching service, helps farmers locate and acquire farmland, and provides business and hands-on technical training, while managing Lampson Brook Agricultural Reserve, a 400-acre publicly owned farmstead. A recent USDA-funded project, Growing New Farmers, works with more than 150 agricultural service organizations to create and improve programs for new farmers throughout the Northeast. One of the directors also serves as the coordinator of the Northeast Sustainable Agriculture Working Group.

I get tired just describing the work of these truly remarkable advocates. Needless to say, our future food situation will be that much brighter, thanks to their efforts.

There are too many groups across the country supporting small-scale farmers to attempt to describe them all. They range from multi-faceted organizations like NESFI to single-purposed specialty programs such as FarmNet. I am most familiar with New York FarmNet, affiliated with Cornell University. Its mission is to provide farm families with a network of contacts and support services to help them develop skills for dealing with significant life challenges and transitions — through personalized education, confidential consulting, and referral. In 2000, NY FarmNet responded to 2,035 calls from the farm community, two-thirds of which were about farm finances and farm stress. It also provided on-farm consultations to 501 farm businesses. As more farm families struggle to stay in business while their neighboring farmers leave the landscape, the need for such a resource is clear.

Growing up, growing food ... urban style

While some children in rural and suburban areas today may have been less exposed to growing food than we might think, youth programs in inner cities are focusing on planting their own gardens. The Food Project in Boston is one of the most successful. The young people, from all socioeconomic levels in the community, work together side by side, running a CSA farm and growing crops to feed low-income families at Friday afternoon lunches in the summer. Another urban project spins the fruits of their youthful labor into salad dressings for sale at local grocery stores. And in Philadelphia, a school market is being developed. Let's learn a little more of their stories.

"**Youth programs in inner cities are focusing on planting their own gardens. The Food Project in Boston is one of the most successful.**"

First, the Food Project. What started as a pilot program nearly a decade ago in Lincoln, Massachusetts, has now become a vibrant hub of activity in multiple locations. According to its website, The Food Project "now boasts a staff of 16, a summer crew of 60 teens (60 percent inner-city, 40 percent suburban), and close to 25 acres of conservation and inner-city land that yield over 200,000 pounds of organic produce annually — 50 kinds of vegetables alone. Over half of the produce goes to 15 Boston food pantries and shelters. An additional 1,000 volunteers donate time in the fields and food lots. One-third of the teens that join in the summer continue in a year-round program ... Two low-cost, inner-city farmers' markets, several small food businesses, a series of free community lunches (prepared by local chefs), a Community Supported Agriculture program, and an EPA-sponsored environmental awareness program have also taken root. Soon the Food Project will open a commercial kitchen in its Dorchester headquarters."[2] The list goes on and on. This expression of "help in the community, by the community" is clearly empowering.

At a recent CSA conference, a handful of teens showed up with farmer Don Zasada to share their experiences in the Food Project. Enthusiastic and dedicated, these youth spread a spirit from the Earth that they seemed to have carried directly from the farm to the conference, a fitting embodiment of this remarkable program.

In 1999, the Food Project and the American Community Gardening Association sponsored the first Rooted in Community conference in Boston, initiating a network, stretching across the US and into Canada, of organizations committed to youth, food, and community. Coordinated by the Food Project, the group provides a newsletter and technical advice, workshops, training, and mini-grants for start-ups.

"Another urban youth program that started in the early 1990s is Food from the Hood in Los Angeles."

Another urban youth program that started in the early 1990s is "Food from the Hood" in Los Angeles. What started as an opportunity to raise food for the homeless in an abandoned garden near the Crenshaw High School has become a profitable food business for student entrepreneurs. The project's employees must maintain a 2.5 grade-point average, and they accumulate shares in the profits based on how many hours they work. The money is paid to graduating seniors in the form of college scholarships.[3] In the summer of 2000, five rotating groups of five students (25 in all) headed to Hanover, Germany, to introduce their brand of salad dressing at the More than Food Expo, part of the World's Fair. The salad dressing brought more than a trip overseas to these students; its sales raised more than $140,000 for scholarships, sending 70 students to college.[4]

School business programs are also emerging. One such program, the School Market Program, has taken hold in Philadelphia-area high schools. Created by the Farmer's Market Trust, the program helps students develop, own, and operate school food markets, selling fruit- and vegetable-related products to fellow students and teachers during the school year. The program's emphasis on food and nutrition learned through application is a wonderful introduction for these students to many of the issues described in this book.

The big picture

Working within urban communities, specifically on hunger and access to safe and nutritious foods, has become a movement within the movement. "Food security" is the term used to describe the issue of equitable distribution of food for all people. One of the most notable organizations engaged in this area is the Hartford Food System in Hartford, Connecticut.

The Hartford Food System (HFS) is a private, non-profit organization established in 1978 to create an equitable and sustainable food system addressing the underlying causes of hunger and poor nutrition faced by lower-income and elderly Connecticut residents. HFS has developed dozens of projects, initiatives, and coalitions that tackle the problems of food cost, access, and nutrition. More recently, it has begun to provide training throughout Connecticut and across the country.

> " Food security is the term used to describe the issue of equitable distribution of food for all people. One of the most notable organizations engaged in this area is the Hartford Food System in Hartford, Connecticut."

The HFS is involved in a never-ending list of activities. From its 168-acre CSA project at the Holcomb Farm, it raises enough food to serve up an annual 3,000 pounds of food to eight Hartford-based community organizations and 300 pounds of food to 200 neighboring households; its grocery delivery service provides affordable food to almost 100 homebound seniors, most of whom live in or near poverty. The HFS is a beehive of sustainable solutions.

There are two things I greatly admire about HFS executive director Mark Winnie and program director Elizabeth Wheeler. First is their willingness to pilot a project and forego its continuation if it doesn't appear as fruitful as hoped. I can think of at least a couple of activities they have tested — a farm-to-school cafeteria program and a farmer-run cooperative retail operation, both of which were eliminated after close evaluation. I also admire their dedication to research. They will commission market studies, poverty and hunger studies, and other pieces of work to inform their decisions, and they will share the information as widely as they can with the local community and with the community of the sustainable agriculture movement. For this, I am grateful.

Mark is also involved with policy work at a national level. He has been instrumental in the formation of a network of organizations devoted to food security — the Food Security Coalition (FSC). The coalition is made up of more than 600 member groups and played a major role in the passage of the 1996 Community Food

Act as part of that year's US Farm Bill. As a result, the USDA has provided $16 million in funding to local food security groups over the past seven years.

The mission of the FSC, a California-based national network, is "to bring about lasting social change by promoting community-based solutions to hunger, poor nutrition, and the globalization of the food system." Activities range from networking diverse organizations, such as anti-hunger groups and environmentalists, information-sharing, farm-to-schools programs, and policy work.

A leading policy-focused organization for the movement is the Henry A. Wallace Center for Agricultural & Environmental Policy at Winrock International, led by Kate Clancy, clearly one of the movement's leaders. The center's mission is "to use its expertise in research, policy analysis, and development to foster sustainable and equitable agricultural and food systems." It does this by providing the leadership, policy research, and analysis necessary to influence national agricultural policy. In addition to a policy studies report series, the center publishes the monthly *Alternative Agriculture News*.

One of its recent contributions is the report "Making Changes: Turning Local Visions into National Solutions: Ninety-five agriculture and rural development policy recommendations developed by the Wallace Center's five-year Agriculture Policy Project." This Kellogg Foundation-funded effort began in 1997. I remember first hearing about the enormous scope of the project in the Wallace offices, which were then outside of Washington, DC. In 16 policy sessions around the country, 350 people participated in "visioning sessions" by addressing key concerns and discussing broad issues. This information fed the work of nine policy advisors, who then began the task of developing policy recommendations that conveyed the desire of the local voices. A uniquely participatory effort toward policy change, the final results are available at the Wallace Center's website, **<www.winrock.org>**.

The organization I think of as synonymous with policy is the Institute of Agriculture and Trade Policy (IATP), headed by Mark Ritchie. Mark's activity level makes some of these other over-achievers look as if they are relaxing!

The IATP was established in 1986, and has undertaken investigation of and involvement in a wide range of topics. Its primary functions, however, fall under the categories of monitoring, analysis and research; education and outreach; training and technical assistance; and coalition-building and international networking.

While researching this book, I was continually coming across yet another study written by, commissioned by, or produced in collaboration with IATP. It also manages listservs on no fewer than 59 different topics.

My first introduction to IATP was through its European Sustainable Agriculture tour, mentioned in other parts of this book. The concept was amazing. Small groups of no more than a dozen sustainable agriculture marketing advocates visited a variety of projects in different European countries and then convened at a university outside Amsterdam to share all the experiences. This information was then translated into a report, and participants returned to their grassroots projects brimming with new possibilities for North America. This is the level of creativity and progressive thinking at IATP.

If you are at all interested in following up on any of the subjects laid out in this eco-foods guide, I heartily recommend a visit to **<www.iatp.org>**. Whatever direction you take from there, I am confident you will be well informed.

There are too many other organizations to mention here. The American Farmland Trust is working to preserve and protect our agricultural lands; the Land Institute has been working for years on an agricultural system based on the ecological stability of the prairie; the Leopold Center is working on solutions to the negative affects of our industrial farming model. And the list goes on and on.

As much as I don't want to sound like a fundraiser, the truth is that many of these organizations are supported by individual contributions. They need your help. And if we hope to have a sustainable plateful for years to come, we need their help even more.

> **"The truth is that many of these organizations are supported by individual contributions. They need your help."**

21

Food for Thought

ECO-EATING IS NO EASY AFFAIR. It takes care and work to make informed decisions. Conflicting values and unfinished research means we just don't know it all. But lots of groups across the country are doing a lot of thinking. Many of the issues in this book lead to value judgments and difficult ethical choices. Do we feed the hungry by developing higher-yielding crops, even if it might harm the Earth? Is good, clean food available to all people or just those wealthy enough to afford the extra cost? Do I have the "right" to purchase GMO foodstuffs for school lunches when I am responsible for other people's children? These are some of the questions being asked in conversations across the country and ones we, ultimately, need to ask ourselves.

Throughout this book we have discussed the importance of our individual decision-making power — the candy-counter syndrome, as named by Paul Thompson, Purdue University ethics professor and agricultural ethics author. Standing in front of the counter as children, we tried to choose between buying one of the candies or saving our money. That decision affected us and, supposedly, the system for candy development. You get the analogy. We make a personal decision and it helps define the "market," not to mention ourselves. We can also act as "food citizens" by taking personal responsibility for shaping our food system. The Wisconsin Foodshed Research Project has defined a food citizen as follows: "Food citizens are eaters who take an interest in food beyond its affordability and availability. Food citizens are concerned about environmental sustainability, the health of farmers and consumers, issues of justice for farmworkers and the poor, and democratic participation in determining where our food system is heading." So if we decide to take on this responsibility, how do we start thinking on a personal level about the ethics and values we have discussed?

"Food citizens are eaters who take an interest in food beyond its affordability and availability. Food citizens are concerned about environmental sustainability, the health of farmers and consumers, issues of justice for farmworkers and the poor, and democratic participation in determining where our food system is heading."

Where to begin?

I am not a particularly religious person, but I am a spiritual being. In my own experience, I have found that when I am right with my personal actions, I feel better … as simple as that. What I have also found is that the different traditions (from Judaism and Christianity to Buddhism and Islam) have lots to share and often agree on ethics and right livelihood.

A wonderful springboard for my own reflection has been the work of Thomas Berry, particularly his alternative worldview, which he calls the New Story. Most of us are anthropocentric, living as if everything revolves around humanity. I love the example given by Sister Miriam McGillis, who speaks on Berry's work, showing how our language reinforces this mindset. For many years now, we have known with the help of Sir Isaac Newton and others that the Earth is actually revolving and spinning itself around the sun. And yet, isn't it true that we still refer to the sunrise as if the sun were to rise on Earth? (An accessible fantasy that can truly reshape our thinking about human-centeredness is the book, *Ishmael* by Daniel Quinn.)

In many of our religious upbringings, the questions about our relationship to food and how it was produced have drawn in part from Bible passages on dominion. "See, I give you every seed-bearing plant all over the earth and every tree that has seed-bearing fruit on it to be your food; and to all the animals of the land, all the birds of the air, and all the living creatures that crawl on the ground, I give all the green plants for food." (Genesis 1, 29–30) So we grow up looking at the Earth as something under our purview. Berry's work goes beyond suggesting improved stewardship, which only reinforces the "power-over" relationship, to suggest we are but a single part of a living, breathing entity known as Earth. This subtle but profound shift readjusts one's thinking on many levels. It suggests that since we are one with the Earth, we are as healthy or as sick as it is. It suggests our collective consciousness is an expression of the Earth, not of individuals living on top of it. This thinking is also expressed in the Buddhist concept of being one with all things, a lack of separation of self.

Mary Evelyn Tucker, one of my heroes — a professor of Theology at Bucknell University who has led thinkers into the confluence of religion and ecology at a series of conferences at Harvard and elsewhere, and who has edited a wonderful book on Buddhism and ecology — describes Berry's work eloquently:

> As Berry has frequently said, there can be no peace among humans without peace with the planet. This, in short, is the intent of the New Story. The underlying assumption is that with a change of worldview will come an appropriately comprehensive ethics of reverence for all life. With a new perspective regarding our place in this extraordinary unfolding of Earth history will emerge a renewed awareness of our role in guiding the evolutionary process at this crucial point in history.
>
> By articulating a new mythic consciousness of our profound connectedness to the Earth we may be able to reverse the self-destructive cultural tendencies we have put in motion with regard to the planet. In so doing we will create the basis for long range economic and ecological sustainability.[1]

How did we get so far off the track? Four centuries ago, Francis Bacon, who has been celebrated as the "father of modern science," was big on discovering nature's secrets, to better manage or constrain her. What can we learn in order to then improve the human life? It was not the discipline of research he advocated that is under scrutiny, but the attitude of dominance and control.

Then, of course, there was Descartes, another founder of modern science, who taught us a mechanistic worldview. Fritjof Capra suggests, "The Cartesian division allowed

"It is tough to respect the earth when one is trained to see it as a big machine."

scientists to treat matter as dead and completely separate from themselves, and to see the world as a multitude of different objects assembled into a huge machine."[2] It is tough to respect the earth when one is trained to see it as a big machine. The mechanistic view just doesn't look at the relationships between things, but sticks safely to the separate parts. Quantum physics refutes this view, but we are still stuck with a reductionist mentality … reduce things to formal logic and explain how the whole works within this model.

Why is this a problem for agriculture? Because as we try to control, manipulate, and explain away, the less we need to believe that there is a miracle in the making of our food. As John Ikerd of the University of Missouri puts it, "The more we understood about the working of the universe, the less we needed to understand about the nature of God. The more we 'knew' the less we needed to 'believe.' As we expanded the realm of the 'factual' we reduced the realm of the 'spiritual' until it became trivial, at least in matters of science."

I would also add that the more we seem to understand nature, the more capable we seem to be of messing it up. I remember listening to Wes Jackson on a speakerphone as he spoke to plant and soil science faculty from a phone booth somewhere between Kansas and Idaho. (He considered it an important opportunity to share with Land Grant agricultural researchers.) He said, "What makes us think we can do something better, that nature has been doing for 6 billion years?" Having watched human progress since before time, I can only guess how the mountains must be laughing at us now.

Ikerd added, at a recent Soul of Agriculture conference, "When we created industrialized agriculture, we destroyed its soul. We proclaimed a new theology of technology. We thought, 'Who needs God? We have science and technology.' And yet, now this industrial scientific agriculture is in crisis. The root cause is the removal of the respect of life from agriculture."

A variety of disciplines or movements are emerging from this train of thought. One of those is bioethics. As bioethicist Michael W. Fox puts it, "Bioethics posits that all life has been created by forces we do not yet fully comprehend, and that life is ours only in sacred trust. In a highly pragmatic sense, bioethics teaches us that when we take care of the Earth, the Earth will feed us and that when we don't take care of nature, nature cannot take care of us."[3]

Although not directly focused on Earth ethics, ecofeminism is another area where "domination of" versus "relationship with" the Earth is central to the discussion. From the website **<www.ecofem.org>**:"Ecofeminism is the social movement that regards the oppression of women and nature as interconnected. It is one of the few movements and analyses that actually connects two movements. More recently, ecofeminist theorists have extended their analyses to consider the interconnections between sexism, the domination of nature (including animals), and also racism and social inequalities. Consequently it is now better understood as a movement working against the interconnected oppressions of gender, race, class and nature."[4]

Back to food and a statement from *Coming into the Foodshed.* "It is through food that humanity's most intimate and essential connections to the Earth and to other creatures are expressed and consummated."[5]

Scholars study agricultural values and ethics

Entire academic associations have been developed to give some outlet for these ideas. In the US, one is the Agriculture, Food and Human Values Society (AFHVS). Founded in 1987, AFHVS promotes interaction between liberal arts and agricultural disciplines, providing a continuing link among scholars working in cross-disciplinary studies of food and agriculture. AFHVS provides a forum for examining the values that underlie various visions of food and agricultural systems, and it offers members opportunities to meet and discuss programs and research ideas of common interest. In her 1996 presidential address to the organization, Kate Clancy refers to the organization's *raison d'être* as follows: "[Paul] Thompson reflects at one point … that 'nearly gone is the spirit of raising food and eating it as an act of communion with the larger whole'. An articulated ethic that helps us and our fellow citizens recover that spirit is what I think we would be well to be about."[6] Paul Thompson is the same ethics professor mentioned earlier in reference to his candy counter analogy. His book *Spirit of the Soil*, published in 1995, has had a great influence on the scholarly, as well as practical, application of combining ethics and agriculture.

Another newer organization is evolving in Europe with some involvement of groups from North America. EurSafe, the European Society for Agricultural and Food Ethics was founded in 1999 and aims to encourage academic education, research, and international debate on the ethical issues involved in agriculture and food supply. The network holds annual conferences and produces publications for furthering the group's aims.

Faith-based groups focus on agricultural ethics

Earth Ministry is a Christian ecumenical, environmental non-profit organization based in Seattle. It was born in 1992 out of recognition of the underlying spiritual and moral roots of the environmental crisis, and the desire to help people of faith see more clearly the connections between their faith, their daily lives, and ecological concerns.

241

Although their purpose is much larger in scope, they do provide a variety of educational materials focusing on individual responsibility with food, such as *Food, Faith and Sustainability: Environmental, Spiritual, Community, and Social Justice Implications of the Gift of Daily Bread*, a five-session book/curriculum guide that "will encourage movement from passive consumerism to mindful participation in all the systems involved in bringing food from farmer to table."

A number of faith-based organizations provide information and resources to readers of their websites, who can then converse with other members of their communities, synagogues, and parishes. One of these is the Web of Creation **<www.webofcreation.org>**, established to facilitate personal and social transformation to a just and sustainable world from religious perspectives. It is maintained by the Lutheran School of Theology at Chicago and is supported by organizations such as the Eco-Justice Working Group of the National Council of Churches, Theological Education to Meet the Environmental Challenge, Evangelical Lutheran Church in America, and the Presbyterian Church.

The Coalition on the Environment and Jewish Life (COEJL) was founded in 1993 to promote environmental education, scholarship, advocacy, and action in the American Jewish community. COEJL is the Jewish member of the National Religious Partnership for the Environment. On their website, they encourage readers to take action to understand the ecology of their food and to choose behaviors encouraging a healthy Earth **<www.coejl.org>**.

The North American Coalition for Christianity and Ecology (NACCE) is an ecumenical organization established in 1986 to encourage the many strands of Christian tradition in the work of healing the damaged Earth, from a common concern and love for God's creation, and to address effectively the greatest moral issue of our time: our continuing destruction of the Earth. Its newsletter, "Earthkeeping News," provides some interesting information.

Another organization providing a series of church bulletin inserts is the National Catholic Rural Life Conference. Its "Ethics of Eating" cards are available as part of the "Eating is a Moral Act" campaign. The source of the campaign is a coalition formed initially to focus on the 2001 Farm Bill, including NCRLC, the National Family Farm Coalition, and the National Campaign for Sustainable Agriculture. The campaign reaches out to the "eaters" of the world, focusing on the moral dimension of the food system. NCRLC has sold thousands of the cards since they became

"The National Catholic Rural Life Conference's Ethics of Eating cards are available as part of the Eating is a Moral Act campaign."

available in 2000. NCRLC is also running a "Green Ribbon" campaign, asking people to wear one to show their solidarity with farm families suffering distress related to the current food-system crisis.

There are surely a multitude of great materials being produced by faith-based and partner organizations. Those I mention above are the most notable of which I am aware. One other that deserves notice is one of the best and most comprehensive documents out there for congregational involvement for sustainable agriculture. The publication *To Till and Keep It* was put together by Dan Guenthner as part of a joint project of the Evangelical Lutheran Church in America and the Land Stewardship Project. After a paper on a particular sustainable agriculture issue, the materials answer the question, "What can we do to respond to the needs of the land?" with very practical and useful suggestions for action.

Finally, a quiet movement to transform more of our land to viable agricultural operations in right relation to a higher power is afoot amongst the Roman Catholic nuns of North America. Sisters of Earth, a network of Roman Catholic religious women and affiliated laity, are converting their land and institutions into centers of ecological literacy and environmental sustainability.[7] Jesuit Al Fritsch at Appalachia Science in the Public Interest has been instrumental in the Sisters of Earth movement by conducting resource audits of their lands to improve food self-reliance and sustainability. Based on these audits, the sisters have reshaped their operations.[8] Many of the sisters have integrated Earth-based literacy based on the work of Thomas Berry. The most important center is Genesis Farm in Blairstown, New Jersey, where Sister Miriam McGillis lives and shares her interpretations of Berry's work. Founded in 1980 by the Dominican Sisters of Caldwell, New Jersey, the 226-acre setting features a working CSA farm as well as a curriculum of Earth literacy offerings, from day-long events to a 12-week college credit course.

Soul of agriculture

Early in 1996, a group of farmers and others concerned about the future of agriculture were struck by Paul Thompson's book *Spirit of the Soil*. The resulting Soul of Agriculture project was initiated in March 1997, from a three-day drafting meeting with more than 20 farmers, faith community representatives, environmentalists, academics, and others. They produced a *Vision Statement/Call to Action: Building a New Ethic of Production in Agriculture*. The Center for Respect of Life and Environment, and the Humane Society of the United States were the original supporters in this attempt to stimulate national discussion about ethical approaches to agricultural production.

The first draft, which included four specific tasks, was presented to more than 200 participants at a Soul of Agriculture national conference held in Minneapolis, Minnesota, in November 1997. As the keynote speaker at that conference, Paul Thompson said, "We need a production ethic for agriculture in which we are all producers, one in which we come to understand ourselves as partners with nature in reproducing the social and ecological environment where our children will themselves face the challenges of production and reproduction."[9]

After a period of disseminating the Soul of Agriculture information, a renewed effort began in the fall of 2001, with a conference held at the University of New Hampshire, again with the support of the Center for Life and Respect for the Environment. There, the ethics expanded outside the farm gate to include all of us — the food citizens. Today the Soul of Agriculture project exists to continue the dialogue with all of u;, from farmer to CSA member, from nutritionist to the family cook.

We all need to be engaged in this movement, no matter from where the spiritual connection comes. It is up to us. We are the producers of our own fare by acting as decision-makers. No matter how we look at it, every moment we ingest another morsel, it reflects a choice we have made. It is either good for the Earth and all its beings, or not.

Of course, we are all humans, struggling to squeeze a whole meal into a fraction of time. We aren't perfect. As my friend just reminded me in response to my whining, "Lighten up, loosen up, and let go!" We can only do what we can do. And yet, I know I feel best when I have made a personal choice that seems right. When I choose antibiotic-free chicken for pasta, or when I see my son chomping down on an organically grown apple, I feel good. When we run out of milk and have the rBGH version from the local gas station's quick-market, I cringe when the children fill their cereal bowls. I just don't feel good about it.

Will we ever know if the food that is best for the Earth is actually scientifically proven to be good for us? The debate will probably continue for a long time. Has it ever been scientifically proven that when we do something loving and caring for another person instead of ourselves, it is actually good for us?

We have been given a gift, although on some days, in our over-committed lifestyles, food feels much more like a chore than a gift. But still and all, it feels good to say thank you. I can do that best by being a food steward: by caring about what happens to the source from which our food comes, and by choosing food that has been raised with fairness to all people and sentient beings. I can choose eco-foods simply because what is good for me is good for the Earth; and what is good for the Earth is good for me.

> "It feels good to say thank you. I can do that best by being a food steward: by caring about what happens to the source from which our food comes, and by choosing food that has been raised with fairness to all people and sentient beings."

Endnotes

Introduction

1. Frances Moore Lappé, *Diet for a Small Planet, Twentieth Anniversary Edition* (Ballantine Books, 1991), p. 12.
2. David Wann, "Organic Farmers Forge Links with Consumers," *Denver Post* (November 25, 2001).

Chapter 1 Shopping for Eco-foods

1. Brewster Kneen, *Farmageddon* (New Society Publishers, 1999), p. 190.

Chapter 2 "GMOs, Pesticides, and Drugs, Oh, My!"

1. John Wargo, *Our Children's Toxic Legacy: How Science and Law Fail to Protect us From Pesticides* (Yale University Press, 1996), p.15.
2. Wargo, *Our Children's Toxic Legacy*, p. 162.
3. US Trade Imports, Commodity and Marketing Programs, Foreign Agriculture Service, United States Department of Agriculture 2001.
4. Wargo, *Our Children's Toxic Legacy*, p. 166.
5. Arnold L. Aspelin and Arthur H. Grube, *Pesticides Industry Sales and Usage 1996 and 1997 Market Estimates* (United States Environmental Protection Agency, November, 1999) p. 3.
6. Wargo, *Our Children's Toxic Legacy*, p. 7.
7. "What Have They Done to Our Food?", *60 Minutes II*, CBS News Broadcasts (August 9, 2001).
8. "Harvest of Fear", Jon Palfreman, Frontline/NOVA, Public Broadcasting Service (April 24, 2001).
9. Peter McKenna, "Industry can't be left to Regulate GM foods," *Toronto Star Newspapers* (August 20, 2001), p. A17.
10. David Appell, "The New Uncertainty Principle," *Scientific American* (January, 2001).
11. Stanly W.B. Ewe and Arpad Pusztai, "Effects of diets containing genetically modified potatoes expressing Galanthus nivalis lectin on rat small intestine," *The Lancet*, vol. 354 no. 9187 (October 16, 1999), p. 1353.
12. Margaret Mellon, Charles Benbrook, and Karen Lutz Benbrook, eds., Union of Concerned Scientists, "Hogging It: Estimates of Antimicrobial Abuse in Livestock" (January 2001), p. xii.
13. Ibid., p. xiii.
14. Ibid., p. xii.

Chapter 3 The Earth First

1. Jack Kerrigan and Margaret Nagel, *Ohio State University Master Gardeners Training Manual* [Ohio State University Extension online], [cited April 2002], <http://www.hcs.ohio-state.edu/mg/manual>.
2. Fred Kirschenmann, "On Becoming Lovers of the Soil," in J. Patrick Madden and Scot G. Chaplowe, eds., *For All Generations: Making World Agriculture More Sustainable* (World Sustainable Agriculture Association, 1997), pp. 101–114.
3. Gail Schumann, *Plant Diseases: Their*

Biology and Social Impact (APS Press, 1991), p. 10.

4. Victor Davis Hanson, *The Land Was Everything: Letters from an American Farmer* (The Free Press, 2000), pp. 59-60.

5. Ibid., p. 57.

6. Merrill Ross and Carole Lembi, *Applied Weed Science* (Macmillan Publishing Company, 1985), p.1.

7. Donald Borror, Dwight M. DeLong, and Charles A. Triplehorn, *An Introduction to the Study of Insects* (CBC College Publishing, 1982), p. 1.

8. Smithsonian National Museum of Natural History, Department of Systematic Biology Entomology [online], (last updated 4/6/2001) [cited February 2002], <www.entomology.si.edu>.

Chapter 4 How We Got Here from There

1. Paul Bonnifield, *The Dust Bowl: Men, Dirt and Depression* (University of New Mexico Press, 1979).

2. "Surviving the Dust Bowl," *The American Experience*, Chana Gazit, Public Broadcasting Service/WGBH Educational Foundation (©1998).

3. John R. Wunder, Francis W. Kaye, and Vernon Carstensen, *Americans View Their Dust Bowl Experience* (University Press of Colorado, 1999), p. 356.

4. "Surviving the Dust Bowl," *The American Experience*, Chana Gazit, PBS.

5. Wunder, Kaye, and Carstensen, *Americans View Their Dust Bowl Experience*, p. 358.

6. Ibid., p. 358.

7. R. Douglas Hurt, *The Dust Bowl: An Agricultural and Social History* (Nelson-Hall, 1981), p. 53.

8. "Surviving the Dust Bowl," *The American Experience*, Chana Gazit, PBS.

9. Wunder, Kaye, and Carstensen, *Americans View Their Dust Bowl Experience*, p. 352.

10. Gregg Easterbrook, "Forgotten benefactor of humanity," *The Atlantic Monthly* (January 1997), p. 74.

11. Vaclav Smil, *Feeding the World: A Challenge for the Twenty-first Century* (MIT Press, 2000).

12. Vandana Shiva, "The Green Revolution in the Punjab," *The Ecologist*, vol. 21, no. 2 (March/April 1991).

13. USDA/NASS, *Trends in US Agriculture: A 20th Century Time Capsule* [online],[cited April 2002], <www.usda.gov/nass/pubs/trends/index.htm>.

14. Peter M. Rosset and Miguel A. Altieri, "Agroecology versus Input Substitution: A Fundamental Contradiction of Sustainable Agriculture," *Society & Natural Resources*, vol. 10 (1997), p. 284.

15. Ibid., p. 287.

16. John Ikerd, "Sustainable Agriculture: A Positive Alternative to Industrial Agriculture," Presentation at the Heartland Roundup in Manhattan, KS (December 7, 1996).

17. William Greider, "The Last Farm Crisis: the New Politics of Food," *The Nation* (November 20, 2000).

18. William D. Heffernan, "Concentration of Ownership and Control in Agriculture," in Fred Magdoff, John

Bellamy Foster, and Frederick H. Buttel, eds., *Hungry for Profit: The Agribusiness Threat to Farmers, Food and the Environment* (Monthly Review Press, 2000), p. 66.

19. Greider, "The Last Farm Crisis: the New Politics of Food."

20. Ibid.

21. Elizabeth Becker, "Land Rich in Subsidies, and Poor in Much Else," *The New York Times* (January 22, 2002), p. 14.

22. Ibid.

23. John Lancaster, "More Subsidy Money Going to Fewer Farms; Skewed Program Draws Senate Scrutiny," *The Washington Post* (January 24, 2002).

24. Geoffrey Becker, "Farm Commodity Programs: A Short Primer," *Congressional Research Service Report for Congress* (September 14, 2001).

25. USDA, "Food and Agriculture Policy — Taking Stock for the New Century," p. 49.

26. Lancaster, "More Subsidy Money…"

27. Geoffrey Becker, "Farm Commodity Programs."

28 Ibid.

Chapter 5 The Great and Powerful Consumer

1. Donella Meadows, "Consumer Power Reforms Chicken Factories — But Not Enough," *The Global Citizen* (September 28, 2000).

2. Cameron Woodwoth, "GMOs: A Growing Concern," *Health Products Business* (October 1999), p. 34.

3. Liz Allen, "Most Land-Grant Schools Slight Organics," *World-Herald*, Omaha, NE (April 22, 2001).

4. Lawrence C. Soley, *Leasing the Ivory Tower: The Corporate Takeover of Academia* (South End Press, 1995).

5. Alice Cooper, *Bitter Harvest* (Routledge, 2000), pp.148–149.

6. Elizabeth Henderson, "Rebuilding local food systems from the grassroots up" in Fred Magdoff, Jeremy Foster, and Frederick Buttel, eds., *Hungry for Profit: The Agribusiness Threat to Farmers, Food and the Environment* (Monthly Review Press, 2000), p.186.

Chapter 6 Don't Worry, Buy Local

1. Kate Clancy, "Regionalism to Nationalism … and Back?" *Northeast Sustainable Agriculture Working Group Resource Harvest White Papers* (Northeast Sustainable Agriculture Working Group, 1998), p. 1.

2. Mary Hendrickson, William D. Heffernan, Philio H. Howard, and Judith B. Heffernan, "Consolidation in Food Retailing and Dairy: Implications of Farmers and Consumers in a Global Food Society," *Report to the National Farmers Union* (January 8, 2001).

3. Joan Dye Gussow, "Keeping Farmers (and Yourself) Alive," *Why* (Fall/Winter 1997), p. 44.

4. Ibid., p. 44

5. Gary Valen, "Eating with Conscience is Good for You and Your Community," *Why* (Fall/Winter 1997), p. 28.

6. Alan Durning, "How Much is Enough?" The WorldWatch Environmental Alert Series (W.W. Norton & Company, 1992), p.73.

7. Ibid.

8. The Cornucopia Project of Rodale Press, *Empty Breadbasket? The Coming*

Challenge to America's Food Supply and What We Can Do About It (Rodale Press, 1981), p.29.

9. Ibid.

10. Ibid.

11. Michael Shumann, "Amazing Shrinking Machines: The Planning Implications of Diminishing Economies of Scale," (unpublished article, 2000).

12. Jack Kloppenburg, Jr., John Henrickson, and G.W. Stevenson, "Coming into the Foodshed," *Agriculture and Human Values*, vol. 14, no. 2 (June 1997), p. 113.

13. Shumann, "Amazing Shrinking Machines."

14. Julia Freedgood, American Farmland Trust, "Paradise Paved," *Northeast Sustainable Agriculture Working Group Resource Harvest White Papers* (Northeast Sustainable Agriculture Working Group, 1998).

15. Douglas J. Krieger, "Saving Open Spaces: Public Support for Farmland Protection," American Farmland Trust's Center for Agriculture in the Environment (April 1999), p. 3.

16. Elizabeth Henderson, "Northeast Food System Analysis" *Northeast Sustainable Agriculture Working Group Resource Harvest White Papers* (Northeast Sustainable Agriculture Working Group, 1998).

17. Shumann, "Amazing Shrinking Machines."

18. Shumann, "Amazing Shrinking Machines."

19. Fred Kirschenmann, "Rebuilding Rural Communities," *Biodynamics* (January/February 1997).

20. John M. Gowdy and Carl N. McDaniel, "The Physical Destruction of Nauru: An Example of Weak Sustainability," *Land Economics*, vol. 75, no. 2 (May 1999), p. 333.

21. Mark Mulcahy, "From Down the Road or Across the Sea, Produce Tells Tales," *Natural Foods Merchandiser* (May 2000).

22. Warren Leon, "Eating for the Environment," *Conservation Matters* (Summer 2000), p. 15.

23. Jennifer Yezak Molen, Barbara Meister, and Cheryl Delamater, "A Time to Act: A Report of the USDA National Commission on Small Farms," (USDA, January 1998).

24. Molly Anderson, "The Politics of the Plate," *Conservation Matters* (Summer 2000), p. 10.

25. Community Involved in Sustaining Agriculture [online], (November 2000), [cited March 2002], <www.buylocalfood.com>.

Chapter 7 'Tis the Season

1. Terra Brockman, "Lettuce Pray," *Conscious Choice* (May 2000).

2. Fran McManus, review of "Cooking Fresh from the Bay Area," The Book Stall, Farmer's Market [online], (2002), [cited March 2002], <www.farmersmarketonline.com/aboutus.htm>.

3. Laura B. DeLind, "Local Food — Overcoming the Distance," *Synapse* (Summer 1997).

4. Rich Pirog, Timothy Van Pelt, Kamyar Enshayan, and Ellen Cook, Leopold Center for Sustainable Agriculture, "Food, fuel and freeways," (June 2001)

5. Joan Dye Gussow, "Is Local vs. Global the Next Environmental Imperative?" *Nutrition Today*, vol. 35 (January 2000), p. 29.

6. Brockman, "Lettuce Pray," *Conscious Choice* (May 2000).

7. Deborah Byrd, "Seasons Provide a Fresh Look at Food," *Contra Costa Times* (January 2, 2000).

8. J.L. Wilkins, J.C. Bokaer-Smith, and D. Hilchey, "Local Foods and Local Agriculture — A Survey of Attitudes Among Northeastern Consumers," *Project Report, Division of Nutritional Sciences* (Cornell Cooperative Extension, 1996).

9. Gussow, "Is Local vs. Global the Next Environmental Imperative?"

10. J.L. Wilkins and J.D. Gussow, "Regional Dietary Guidance: Is the Northeast Nutritionally Complete?" *Proceedings of the International Conference on Agricultural Production and Nutrition* (March 19–21, 1997).

11. Laura Fraser, "Homegrown Harvest," *Health*, vol. 11, no. 4 (May-June 1997), p. 70.

12. Iowa State University Extension News and Reports, "Dietary Guidelines for Sustainability" (September 17, 1999).

13. Linda Halley, *Seasonal Eating: A Menu throughout the Year* (Harmony Valley Farm, 2000).

14. Wendy Rickard and Fran McManus, *Cooking Fresh from the Bay Area* (Eating Fresh Publications, 2000).

15. Christina Waters, "Market Value," *Metro* (May 9, 1996).

16. Ibid.

17. Jennifer Wolcott, "Why Real Cooks Love Farmers' Markets," *The Christian Science Monitor* (June 6, 2001).

18. Diane Peterson, "Home Grown," *The Press Democrat Sonoma* (September 13, 2000).

Chapter 8 You Can't Grow Coffee in Maine

1. Timothy Egan, "'Perfect' Apple Pushed Growers Into Debt," *The New York Times* (November 4, 2000).

2. Agnes Perez, USDA/Economic Research Service, "2001 US Apple Crop Smaller, Prices Likely to Rise," *Agricultural Outlook* (October 2001).

3. John Pirog and John Tyndall, "An Iowa Perspective on Apples and Local Food Systems," *Apple Journal* [online], [cited April 2002], <www.applejournal.com/art001a. htm>.

4. J. L. Wilkins and J. D. Gussow, "Regional Dietary Guidance: Is the Northeast Nutritionally Complete?" *Proceedings of the International Conference on Agricultural Production and Nutrition* (March 19–21, 1997).

5. Ibid.

6. Pirog and Tyndall, "An Iowa Perspective on Apples and Local Food Systems."

7. Eugene Kupferman, "Maturity and Harvest of Apples in New Zealand," *Good Fruit Grower* (November 1996).

8. Glenda Neff, NY Farms, "Buy & Sell Local Produce Works for Independent Grocer" *Great Stuff is Made Locally and Market Research Initiative Online Newsletter*, [cited January 2002], <www.greatstuffmadelocally.org/newsl etter/newsletter.htm>.

9. Annette Larson, "Group Touts Local Apples As Safe Food," *Brattleboro*

Reformer (September 24, 1997), p. 1.

10. Daniele Giovannucci, *Sustainable Coffee Survey of the North American Specialty Coffee Industry*, Specialty Coffee Association of America and the North American Commission for Environmental Cooperation (July 2001), p. 7.

11. Jennifer McLean and Paul D. Rice, "Sustainable Coffee at the Crossroads," *White Paper for the Consumer's Choice Council* (October 15, 1999).

12. Francine Stephens, "Profiles in Sustainable Development Partnerships: The Rainforest Alliance & Ralda Investements," *Rainforest Alliance Newsletter* (November 2001).

13. Laure Waridel, *Coffee with Pleasure: Just Java and World Trade* (Black Rose Books, 2001).

14. Ibid.

15. McLean and Rice, "Sustainable Coffee at the Crossroads."

16. Chris Cobb, "Coffee Crunch," *Ottawa Citizen* (November 25, 2001), [part one.]

17. Ibid., [part two.]

18. Ibid., [part one.]

19. Francine Stephens, "Drinking Certified Coffee: A Way Out of the Global Coffee Crisis," *The Canopy* (A Rainforest Alliance Publication, Fall 2001), p. 1.

20. Rainforest Alliance, "Profiles in Sustainable Development Partnerships: The Rainforest Alliance & Chiquita Brands International, Inc.," (August 2001).

21. Jeffrey Cohn, "The International Flow of Food," *FDA Consumer* (January/February 2001), p. 29.

22. Editorial, "Down on the Farm: NAFTA's Seven-Years War on Farmers and Ranchers in the US, Canada and Mexico," *Public Citizen* (Summer 2001).

23. Bernard Simon, "US-Canada Tomato War Heats Up," *The New York Times* (December 7, 2001), Section W, p. 1.

24. Ralph Nader and Lori Wallach, "GATT, NAFTA, and the Subversion of the Democratic Process," in Jerry Mander and Edward Goldsmith, eds., *The Case Against the Global Economy* (Sierra Club Books, 1996).

25. Wendell Berry, "The Idea of a Local Economy," *Orion* (Winter 2001), p. 36.

26. Waridel, *Coffee with Pleasure: Just Java and World Trade*.

Chapter 9 Conveyor Belt Food

1. Rachel Laudan, "A Plea for Culinary Modernism: Why We Should Love New, Fast, Processed Food," *Gastronomica* (February 2001), p. 41.

2. Betty Parham, "Eating Fresh All Year," *The Atlanta Constitution* (March 29, 2001).

3. T.A. Roberts, C.R. Dillion, and T.J. Siebenmorgen, "The Impact of Food Processing on the US Economy," *Food Technology* (October 1996).

4. US Food and Drug Administration FDA/IFIC, "Food Additives," FDA Brochure (January 1992).

5. Ibid.

6. Center for Science in the Public Interest, "Chemical Cuisine: CSPI's Guide to Food Additives" [online], (2002), [cited March 2002], <www.cspinet.org>.

7. R. Piccioni, "Food Irradiation: Contaminating our Food," *Ecologist*, vol. 18, no. 2 (1988), pp. 48–55, in

Samuel S. Epstein and Wenonah Hauter, "Preventing Pathogenic Food Poisoning: Sanitation not Irradiation," *International Journal of Health Services*, vol. 31, no. 1, (2001), pp. 187–192.

8. D.R. Murray, *Biology of Food Irradiation* (RSP Research Studies Press Ltd., 1990), in Epstein and Hauter, "Preventing Pathogenic Food Poisoning," 2001, pp. 187-192.

9. Laudan, "A Plea for Culinary Modernism."

Chapter 10 Bio(tech) Hazards

1. Roseanne Harper, "Americans Still Don't Know Much About Biotech: Poll," *Supermarket News* (November 26, 2001).

2. Jon Palfreman, Frontline/NOVA, Public Broadcasting Service, "Harvest of Fear" (April 24, 2001).

3. Michael Pollan, "Playing God in the Garden," *New York Times Magazine* (October 25, 1998), p. 44.

4. Brewster Kneen, *Farmageddon: Food and Culture of Biotechnology* (New Society Publishers, 1999), p. 27.

5. Cameron Woodworth, "GMOs: A Growing Concern," *Health Products Business*, vol. 45, no. 10 (October 1999), p. 34.

6. Palfreman, Frontline/NOVA, "Harvest of Fear"

7. Martin Teitel and Kimberly A. Wilson, Council for Responsible Genetics, *Genetically Engineered Food: Changing the Nature of Nature* (Park Street Press, 1999), p. 12.

8. Pollan, "Playing God in the Garden," p. 44.

9. Palfreman, Frontline/NOVA, "Harvest of Fear"

10. Kneen, *Farmageddon*, p. 140.

11. Lowell Tickner, Carolyn Raffensperger, and Nancy Myers, *The Precautionary Principle in Action: A Handbook* (Science and Environmental Health Network) [online], [cited April 2002], p. 2, <www. biotech-info.net/handbook.pdf>.

12. Peter Montague, "The Precautionary Principle," *Rachel's Environment and Health Weekly*, no. 586 (February 19, 1998).

13. Craig Holdredge and Steve Talbott, "Sowing Technology: The Ecological Argument Against Genetic Engineering Down on the Farm," *Sierra* (July/August 2001), p. 37.

14. Lincoln P. Brower, "Canary in the Cornfield: the Monarch and the Bt Corn Controversy," *Orion* (Spring 2001), pp. 37–40.

15. Kneen, *Farmageddon*, pp. 114–115.

16. Miguel A. Altieri, "Ten Reasons Why Biotechnology Will Not Ensure Food Security, Protect the Environment or Reduce Poverty in the Developing World," *Food First/Institute for Food and Development Policy* (October 1999).

17. Pollan, "Playing God in the Garden," p. 44.

18. Teitel and Wilson, *Genetically Engineered Food*, p. 95.

19. Sharon Schmickle, "Backlash in Japan Against GM Crops Has Midwest Farmers Worried," *Star Tribune* (April 30, 2000).

20. Michael Pollan, "The Year in Ideas: A to Z: genetic pollution," *The New York Times* (December 9, 2001), p. 74.

21. Mark Stevenson, "Mexicans Angered by Spread of Corn," *Associated Press* (December 29, 2001).

22. Kneen, *Farmageddon*, p. 13.

23. Nic Paget-Clarke, "An Interview with Vandana Shiva," *Motion* (August 14, 1998).

24. Rob Edwards, "End of the Germ Line," *New Scientist* (March 28, 1998).

25. Ann Cooper and Lisa M. Holmes, *Bitter Harvest* (Routledge, 2000), p. 96.

26. Edwards, "End of the Germ Line."

27. Scott Kilman, "High Court Says Seeds Can Be Patented, In Ruling Beneficial to Biotech Industry," *The Wall Street Journal* (December 11, 2001).

28. Teitel and Wilson, *Genetically Engineered Food*, p. xiii.

29. Mark A. Pollack and Gregory Shaffer, "Biotechnology: The Next Transatlantic Trade War?" *The Washington Quarterly*, vol. 23, no. 4 (Autumn 2000), p. 41.

30. Teitel and Wilson, *Engineered Food* p. 91–92.

31. Kneen, *Farmageddon*, p. 29.

32. Brian Halweil, "The Emperor's New Crops, " *World Watch* (July/August 1999).

33. Vandana Shiva, BBC Reith 2000 Lecture Series, BBC Radio (May 10, 2000).

34. Bill Lambrecht, *Dinner at the New Gene Café* (St. Martin's Press, 2001).

35. Michael Pollan, "The Great Yellow Hype," *The New York Times* (March 4, 2001).

36. Ibid.

37. Justin Gillis, "Biotech Firms Launch Food Ad Blitz," *The Washington Post* (April 4, 2000), Section E, p. 1.

38. Teitel and Wilson, *Genetically Engineered Food*, p. 49.

39. Teitel and Wilson, *Genetically Engineered Food*, p. 70.

40. Kneen, *Farmageddon*, p. 144.

41. David Barboza, "As Biotech Crops Multiply, Consumers Get Little Choice," *The New York Times* (June 10, 2001).

42. Julianne Johnston, "2001 Global GM Crop Area Grew to 130 Mil. Acres" [online], (January 10, 2002), <www.agweb.com/>.

43. "What Have They Done to Our Food?" *60 Minutes II*, CBS News Broadcasts (August 9, 2001).

44. Altieri, "Ten reasons why biotechnology…"

45. Pollan, "Playing God in the Garden," p. 44.

46. "State Legislative Activity in 2001 Related to Agricultural Biotechnology," (*Pew Initiative on Food and Biotechnology*), (January 2002).

47. Mia Stainsby, "Food for Thought: John Robbins Warns on GM Foods," *The Vancouver Sun* (January 7, 2002).

48. Scott Kilman, "FDA Warns of Misleading Labels on Genetic Modification in Foods, " *The Wall Street Journal* (December 20, 2001).

Chapter 11 All Creatures Great and Small

1. Leora Vestel and Broydo Vestel, "The Next Pig Thing," *Mother Jones* (October 26, 2001).

2. Melanie Adcock, "The Real Price of Factory Farming," *Wildlife Tracks* (Winter 1998).

3. John Robbins, *The Food Revolution: How Your Diet Can Help Save Your Life*

and the World (Conari Press, 2001), p. 182.

4. Editorial, "Unnatural Lives," *Orion* (Winter 2001), p. 1.

5. Donella Meadows, "Consumer Power Reforms Chicken Factories — But Not Enough," *The Global Citizen* (September 28, 2000).

6. Humane Society of the United States, "Chickens Under Contract: The US Broiler Industry Today," Farm Animals & Sustainable Agriculture Section, (August 1997, updated February 1998).

7. Farm Aid Facts <www.farmaid.org/event/info/faq.asp>.

8. Melanie Adcock, "The Truth Behind 'A Hen's Life,'" *Humane Society of the United States News* (Spring 1993).

9. Ibid.

10. Robbins, *The Food Revolution*, p. 179.

11. Michael Appleby, personal communication (April 2002).

12. Marlene Halverson, *The Price We Pay for Corporate Hogs*, Institute of Agriculture and Trade Policy, July 2000, section 2, p. 3.

13. Christine Gorman, "Playing Chicken With Our Antibiotics: Overtreatment is creating dangerously resistant germs," *Time* (January 21, 2002), p. 98.

14. Ibid., p. 98.

15. "Public-Interest Groups Call on Bayer to Support FDA Ban on Antibiotic Used in Poultry Production," Environmental Defense Press Release (October 31, 2000).

16. Halverson, *The Price We Pay for Corporate Hogs*, section 2, p. 6.

17. Ibid., section 2, p. 4.

18. Melanie Adcock and Mary Finelli, "Against Nature: The Sensitive Pig versus the Hostile Environment of the Modern Pig Farm," *Humane Society of the United States News* (Spring 1996).

19. Robert F. Kennedy Jr., ed., "National Gathering Calls for Humane, Sustainable Hog Farming," *Animal Welfare Institute Quarterly*, vol. 50, no. 1 (Winter 2001).

20. Halverson, *The Price We Pay for Corporate Hogs*, executive summary p. 2.

21. Ibid., section 1, p. 3.

22. Ibid., section 1, p. 3.

23. National Resources Defense Council, "Facts about Pollution from Livestock Farms," *Natural Resources Defense Council Fact Sheet*.

24. Halverson, *The Price We Pay for Corporate Hogs*, section 2, p. 4.

25. National Resources Defense Council, "Facts about Pollution from Livestock Farms."

26. Ibid.

27. Halverson, *The Price We Pay for Corporate Hogs*, section 3, p. 4.

28. Dirk Johnson, "Growth of Factory-like Hog Farms Divides Rural Areas of the Midwest," *The New York Times* (June 24, 1998), section A, p. 12.

29. Gail Collins, "Public Interests: the Pig Wars," *The New York Times* (January 12, 2001), section A, p. 23.

30. Halverson, *The Price We Pay for Corporate Hogs*, section 3, p. 6.

31. Elizabeth Becker, "Unpopular Fee Makes Activists Out of Farmers," *The New York Times* (June 11, 2001).

32. Claude Fischler, "The Mad Cow Crisis: A Global Perspective," in Raymond Grew, ed., *Food in Global History* (Westview Press, 1999), pp. 207–213.

33. Elizabeth Becker, "US Mad Cow Risk Is Low, A Study by Harvard Finds," *The New York Times* (December 1, 2001).

34. Robbins, *The Food Revolution*, p. 206.

35. Melanie Adcock, "The Dairy Cow: America's Foster Mother," *Humane Society of the United States News* (Winter 1995).

Chapter 12 A Fishy Story

1. Peter Montague, "Oceans Without Fish," *Rachel's Environment and Health Weekly* no. 587 (February 26, 1998).

2. Susan Pollack, "City by the Sea" (Winter 2001), pp. 38–45.

3. Monterey Bay Aquarium [online], (2000), [cited March 2002], <www.mbayaq.org>.

4. Francine Stephens, "Seafood Solutions: A Chef's Guide to Ecologically Responsible Fish Procurement," (Chef's Collaborative with Environmental Defense Fund, 2000), p. 2.

5. Steve Nadis, "In Search of Guilt-Free Seafood," *National Wildlife* (December/January 2001).

6. Rebecca J. Goldburg, Matthew S. Elliot, and Rosamund L. Naylor, *Marine Aquaculture in the United States: Environmental Impacts and Policy Options* (Pew Oceans Commission, 2001), p. 2.

7. Ibid., p. 1.

8. Ibid., p. 2.

9. Ibid., p. 18.

10. Bruce Barcott, "Aquaculture's Troubled Harvest," *Mother Jones* (November/December 2001).

11. Goldburg et al., *Marine Aquaculture*, p. 4.

12. Barcott, "Aquaculture's Troubled Harvest."

13. Goldburg et al., *Marine Aquaculture*, p. 7.

14. Ibid., p. 6.

15. Barcott, "Aquaculture's Troubled Harvest."

16. Ibid.

17. Goldburg et al., *Marine Aquaculture*, p. 13.

18. Ibid., p. 14.

19. Anne Platt McGinn, "Blue Revolution: The Promises and Pitfalls of Fish Farming," *WorldWatch*, vol. 14 (March/April 1998), pp. 11–19.

20. Ibid., p. 14.

21. Carol Lewis, "A New Kind of Fish Story: The Coming of Biotech Animals," *FDA Consumer* (January-February 2001), p. 5.

22. Susan Bourette, "The Gene Pool: Aqua Bounty Farms Says Its Genetically Modified Salmon Could Replenish Dwindling Stocks and Salvage the Aquaculture Industry. Environmentalists, scientists and conventional salmon farmers think the company's telling a whopper." *National Post Business Magazine*, vol. 53 (January 1, 2002).

23. Tony Riechhardt, "Will Souped Up Salmon Sink or Swim?," *Nature*, vol 406 (July 6, 2000), pp. 10–12.

24. The Campaign to Label Genetically Engineered Foods, "Blue Revolution Coming as Scientists Develop Genetically Engineered Fish," *Take Action Kit*, (2001), p. 20.

25. Jan Van Aken, "Genetically Engineered Fish: Swimming Against the Tide of Reason," *Biosafety Protocol*, Greenpeace International (January 2000).

26. CBS News, "Genetic Tinkering For Bigger Catch," (February 14, 2000).

Chapter 13 The Lowdown Behind the Labels

1. J. Emil Morhardt, "ISO 14001 and Agriculture: Opinions of Agricultural Academics, Agricultural Consultants, and ISO 14001 Registrars and Auditors, " *White Paper IATP:* "Adding Value Through Environmental Marketing: Opportunites for Food Producers, Processors and Retailers Conference Proceedings," (December 6–7, 1999).

2. Jonathon Moscatello, "Jonathon Moscatello, The Food Alliance," *Grist Magazine* (May 30, 2001), <www.gristmagazine.com>.

3. University of Wisconsin at Madison, WWF/WPVGA/UWM, Collaboration website project background <http://ipcm.wisc.edu/bioipm/>.

4. Priscilla M. Brooks and Jennifer Jacobus, "Labels for a Green Planet, " Conservation Law Foundation (1997) <www.crlf.org>.

5. Melinda Fulmer, "Eco-labels on Food Called into Question," *Los Angeles Times* (August 26, 2001).

Chapter 14 Organic... What Does It Mean?

1. National Organic Standards Board, Organic Trade Association website [cited January 2002], <www.ota.com>.

2. Editorial, "The True Meaning of 'Organic,'" *Acres USA* (September 1999), p. 24.

3. Grace Gershuny, "The Evolution of Organic," in David Richard and Dorie Byers, eds., *Taste Life! The Organic Choice* (Vital Health Publishing, 1998), p. 158.

4. Ibid., p. 159.

5. Editorial, "The True Meaning of 'Organic.'"

6. Robert Fetter, "Economic Impacts of Alternative Scenarios of Organic Products Regulation," *Senior Honors Thesis*, University of Massachusetts at Amherst (May 1999), p. 3.

7. Peter Hoffman, "Going Organic, Clumsily," *The New York Times* (March 24, 1998).

8. Lee Hochberg, "What's Organic?" MacNeil/Lehrer Newshour transcript (March 23, 1998).

9. Hoffman, "Going Organic, Clumsily."

10. Brian Halweil, "Organic Gold Rush, " *WorldWatch* (May/June 2001), p. 31.

11. Organic Trade Association website 2001 <www.ota.com>.

12. Catherine Lawson, "The Green Food Chain: The Grower, the Retailer, the Server, the Consumer," *The Ottawa Citizen* (October 13, 2001).

13. Halweil, "Organic Gold Rush, " pp. 22–23.

14. Ibid., pp. 22–23.

15. Karen Klonsky and Laura Tourte, "Organic Agricultural Production in the United States: Debates and Directions," *American Journal of Agricultural Economics*, no.5 (1998), p. 1121.

16. John Fetto, "Home on the Organic Range: Consumer Trends Help Save a Fading Piece of America," *American Demographics* (August 1999).

17. Bill Liebhardt, "Get the Facts Straight: Organic Agriculture Yields Are Good," *Organic Farming Research Foundation Information Bulletin*, no. 10, p. 6.

18. Ibid., p. 6.
19. Marc Kaufman, "US Sets 'Organic' Standard," *The Washington Post* (December 21, 2000), section A, p. 1.
20. Mary Brophy Marcus, "Organic Foods offer Peace of Mind — at a Price," *US News & World Report*, vol. 130, no. 2, p. 48.
21. Michael Pollan, "The Organic-Industrial Complex," *New York Times Magazine* (May 14, 2001).
22. Ibid.
23. Eric Brazil, "Organic Farming Sprouting Businesses: Chemical-free Produce Hits the Big Time," *The San Francisco Chronicle* (April 22, 2001).
24. Pollan, "The Organic-Industrial Complex."
25. Editorial, "The True Meaning of 'Organic.'"
26. Gershuny, "The Evolution of Organic," pp. 166–167.
27. Halweil, "Organic Gold Rush," p. 31.

Chapter 15 What Does IPM Mean?
Control Freaks
in the Field

1. Charles M. Benbrook with Edward Groth III, Jean M. Halloran, Michael Hansen, and Sandra Marquardt, *Pest Management at the Crossroads* (Consumers Union, 1996), p. 2.
2. Tom Green, personal communication (January 2002).
3. Benbrook, et al., *Pest Management at the Crossroads*, p. 18.
4. Ibid., p. 186.
5. Bob Holmes, "The Joy Ride Is Over," *US News & World Report*, vol. 113, no. 10, p. 73.
6. Pamela G. Marrone, "Biotechnology and Integrated Pest Management Systems," *National Foundation for IPM Education White Papers* <www.ipm-education.org/white_ papers.html>.
7. Benbrook, et al., *Pest Management at the Crossroads*, p. 13.
8. Don Comis, "Corn Belt Growers Give Area Wide IPM a Try," *Agricultural Research*, vol. 45, no. 10, p. 4.
9. Benbrook, et al., *Pest Management at the Crossroads*, p. 22.
10. Ibid., p. 23.
11. Ibid., p. 24.
12. Larry Walker, "Lodi Growers' Innovative Winegrape Package," *Wines & Vines*, (June 1996), p. 57.
13. Tom Green, personal communication (January 2002).
14. United States General Accounting Office, "Agricultural Pesticides Management Improvements Needed to Further Promote Integrated Pest Management," (*GAO Report 01-815*, August 2001), p. 2.
15. USDA, National Integrated Pest Management Initiative: Backgrounder, [online], [cited April 2002] <www.nysaes.cornell.edu/ipmnet/init. bckground.html>.
16. US GAO, "Agricultural Pesticides Management Improvements Needed...," p. 7.
17. Benbrook, et al., *Pest Management at the Crossroads*, p. 196.
18. Gary Gardner, "IPM and the War on Pests," *WorldWatch* (March/April 1996), p. 24.
19. US GAO, "Agricultural Pesticides Management Improvements Needed...," p. 2.

20. Benbrook, et al., *Pest Management at the Crossroads*, p. 27.

Chapter 16 Shopping Alternatives

1. Grant Ferrier, "Sifting Through The Numbers," *Natural Foods Merchandiser* (December 2001).

2. United States Department of Agriculture, Agricultural Marketing Service, "Farmers Market Facts!" [online], (updated June 2001), [cited March 2002], <www.ams.usda.gov/farmersmarkets/facts.htm>.

3. Robert Chorney, "Farmers' Market Ontario History" [online], (January 20, 2001) [cited April 2002], <www.fmo.reach.net/history.html>.

Chapter 17 If You Can't Beat 'em, Join 'em

1. Alan Bisbort, "Saving the Farm through Cooperation," *The New York Times* (April 16, 2000).

2. Robyn VanEn, "Basic Formula to Create Community Supported Agriculture" (Great Barrington, MA, 1992), p. 57.

3. Jim Sluyter and Jo Meller, eds., "Five Springs Farm," *The Community Farm* (Spring 1998).

4. Jim Sluyter and Jo Meller, eds., "More Than Just Veggies," *The Community Farm* (Summer 2001).

5. Ibid.

6. Jack P. Cooley, "Community Supported Agriculture: A Study of Shareholders' Dietary Patterns, Food Practices, and Perceptions of Farm Membership," Masters Thesis, University of Massachusetts (September 1996).

7. Jane M. Kolodinsky and Leslie L. Pelch, "Factors Influencing the Decision to Join a Community Supported Agriculture (CSA) Farm," *Journal of Sustainable Agriculture*, vol. 10, pp. 129–141.

8. Paul Fieldhouse, "Community Shared Agriculture," *Agriculture and Human Values*, vol. 13, no. 3, p. 46.

9. Ibid., p. 123.

10. David Wann, "Organic Farmers Forge Links with Consumers," *Denver Post* (November 25, 2001).

11. Sarah Milstein, "Creating a Market: Getting Started in Community Supported Agriculture," *Mother Earth News*, no. 172.

12. Ruth Katz, personal communication (April 2002).

13. Doug Wubben, "Just Eating," *Madison Area Community Supported Agriculture Coalition Newsletter*, (Summer/Fall 20001), p. 3.

14. Bisbort, "Saving the Farm through Cooperation."

15. Gary Lamb, "Community Supported Agriculture: Can it become the basis for a new associative economy?" *The Threefold Review*, no.11, p. 40.

Chapter 18 Who's Got Time to Cook?

1. Annie Berthold-Bond and Mothers & Others for a Livable Planet, *The Green Kitchen Handbook* (Harper Perennial 1997), p. xix.

2. Editorial, "The Philosophy," *GlobalChefs* [online], (2001), <www.globalchefs.com>.

3. Nancy Civetta, *Chefs Collaborative Fact Sheet* (2001).

4. John Zebrowski, "Chefs Hope To Place Eco-friendly Seafood on Nation's

Menu," *The Seattle Times* (January 21, 2001), section A, p. 1.

5. Ibid., section A, p. 1.

6. Bill Husted, "Chef's Group, Restaurateur Coalition on Verge of Food Fight," *The Denver Post* (February 9, 2001), section EE, p. 6.

7. Earth Pledge website < www.earthpledge.org/>.

8. Editorial, Vermont Fresh Network, *Vermont Fresh Network Dining Guide* (June 2001), p. 2.

9. "Linking Local Chefs and Growers," Gretchen Lehmann, Oregon Public Broadcasting (March 15, 2001).

10. Donna Fenn, "Veggie-Burger Kings" [online], (November 1, 2001), <www.inc.com>.

11. Eric Schlosser, *Fast Food Nation* (Houghton Mifflin Company, 2001), p. 269.

12. Kate Murphy, "Is Healthy Fast Food Leaving a Slow Profit Lane?" *The New York Times* (July 8, 2001).

13. Ibid.

14. John Monahan, "New Fast Foods Offer Healthier Options," *The Natural Foods Merchandiser* (June 2001).

Chapter 19 Your Kids Will Thank You... When They're Older, Maybe

1. Constance L. Hays, "Commercialism in US School Is Examined in New Report," *The New York Times* (September 14, 2000).

2. Shannon Brownlee with Ellen Martins, Jeanne McDowell, and Maggie Sieger, "Too Heavy, Too Young: Obesity is rapidly becoming the major health crisis of the next generation. What parents can do to help kids control their own weight," *Time* (January 21, 2002), p. 88.

3. Ibid., p. 88.

4. United States Department of Agriculture, "Foods Sold in Competition with USDA School Meal Programs," (USDA, January 12, 2001).

5. Eric Schlosser, *Fast Food Nation* (Houghton Mifflin Company, 2001), pp. 218–219.

6. Marion Burros, "US Proposes End to Testing for Salmonella in School Beef," *The New York Times* (April 5, 2001).

7. University of California Agriculture and Natural Resources, "Farm-to-school salad bar program celebrates grand opening" [online], (April 10, 2001), [cited March 2002], <www.oakland.ucanr.org/news/Jan-June2001/saladbar.html>.

8. Susan Lang, "Cornell project will have more local produce in school lunches," *Cornell Chronicle*, vol. 33, no. 2.

9. CNN, "Berkeley Schools Get Taste of Organic Lunch," (September 5, 1999).

10. Laura De Lind, "Interactive Foods for Children: Marketing Child's Play vs. Playing in the Garden," *Gastronomica* (Fall 2001), p. 78.

11. Kristen Markley, "Farm to School/ College Partnerships Subject of December Conference," Cornell University, *Farming Alternatives*, vol. 9, no. 4.

12. Brownlee, et al., "Too Heavy, Too Young," p. 88.

13. Editorial, "Meadowcreek Local Food Project" *Sustainability in Action* (December 1997), p. 15.

14. John E. Carroll, "Greening the Campus," *AboutCampus*, vol 3., no. 6, p. 6.

Chapter 20 People Helping People

1. Fred Magdoff, John Bellamy Foster, and Frederick H. Buttel, *Hungry for Profit: The Agribusiness Threat to Farmers, Food and the Environment* (Monthly Review Press, 2000), p. 175.

2. What Kids Can Do Project Profile, "The Food Project" [online], [cited January 2002], <www.whatkidscando.org/home.htm>

3. Debbie Goldberg, "School Work," *The Washington Post* (October 25, 1998), section R, p. 18.

4. "Crenshaw High Students Take Food Venture to World's Fair," *Los Angeles Times* (June 30, 2000), p. 4.

Chapter 21 Food For Thought

1. Mary Evelyn Tucker, "Thomas Berry and the New Story: An Introduction to the Work of Thomas Berry" [online], Harvard Seminar on Environmental Values website, [cited January 2002], <www.ecoethics.net/ops/tucker.htm>.

2. Fritjof Capra, *Tao of Physics* (Shambhala Publications 1983), p. 22.

3. Michael W. Fox, "Bioethics: Its Scope and Purpose," *Humane Society of the United States News* (Spring 1994).

4. "What is Ecofeminism?" [online], (updated March 3, 2002), [cited March 2002], <www.ecofem.org>.

5. Jack Kloppenburg, Jr., John Henrickson, and G.W. Stevenson, "Coming into the Foodshed," *Agriculture and Human Values*, vol. 13, p. 37.

6. Kate Clancy, "1996 Presidential Address to the Agriculture, Food and Human Values Society," *Agriculture and Human Values*, vol. 14, no. 2, p. 113.

7. Rosemary Radford Ruether, "Sisters of Earth: Religious Women and Ecological Spirituality," *The Witness* (May 2000).

8. Albert J. Fritsch, SJ, *Reflections on Land Stewardship for Religious Communities* (Appalachia — Science in the Public Interest, 2000).

9. Paul Thompson, "A Revitalized Production Ethic for Agriculture," *Earth Ethics* (Spring/Summer 1998), p. 5.

Index